EYE CARE
Netra Jyoti

a text based on our practical Workshop for
HEALTHY VISION, BEAUTIFUL EYES, RELAXED MIND

poses by NANDITA GUPTA
Ashwini Kumar Aggarwal

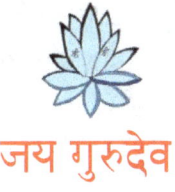

जय गुरुदेव

© 2020, Author

Black/White Plates
ISBN13: 978-81-946008-7-9 Paperback Edition
Full Color Plates
ISBN13: 978-81-946008-8-6 Hardbound Edition
ISBN13: 978-81-946008-9-3 Digital Edition

This work is licensed under a Creative Commons Attribution 4.0 International License. Please visit
https://creativecommons.org/licenses/by/4.0/

Title: **Eye Care Netra Jyoti**
Author: **Ashwini Kumar Aggarwal**

Printed and Published by
Devotees of Sri Sri Ravi Shankar Ashram
34 Sunny Enclave, Devigarh Road,
Patiala 147001, Punjab, India

https://advaita56.weebly.com/
The Art of Living Centre

https://www.artofliving.org/

28th April 2020 Adi Sankara Jayanti, Shukla Paksha Panchami
Skanda Sashti, Grishma Ritu, Uttarayana, Ardra Nakshatra
Vikram Samvat 2077 Pramadi, Saka Era 1942 Sharvari

1st Edition April 2020

जय गुरुदेव

Dedication

Sri Sri Ravi Shankar

His VISION for an Aggression-free Depression-free Society keeps us available, youthful, helpful and caring

Acknowledgements

Dr. Padmalochan Jena of Bangalore Ashram Panchakarma, for excelling in holistic eye care.

Front Cover Photo Credits

Photo by Bess Hamiti from Pexels
https://www.pexels.com/photo/toddle-wearing-gray-button-collared-shirt-with-curly-hair-35537/

Blessing

When we radiate peace and good vibrations, it definitely makes an impact. A bigger VISION of life can kindle human values, enabling one to see diversity in oneness and unity in diversity.

Sri Sri Ravi Shankar
Tweet 8:15 pm Oct 25, 2013 @SriSri

Prayer

ॐ सह नाववतु । सह नौ भुनक्तु । सह वीर्यं करवावहै । तेजस्वि नावधीतमस्तु मा विद्विषावहै ॥ ॐ शान्तिः शान्तिः शान्तिः ॥

oṃ saha nāvavatu | saha nau bhunaktu | saha vīryaṃ karavāvahai | tejasvi nāvadhītamastu mā vidviṣāvahai || oṃ śānti śāntiḥ ||

Peace Invocation
O Pure Loving Grace!

May we be taken care of along with our family and friends.
May we enjoy socializing and eating together.
May we support each other's VISION and growth.
May our intellect be open to new ideas and changing trends.
May we spend more time in praise than abuse, may we talk of each other's virtues rather than harp on vices.

Peace in our heart, in our body, and in our environs.

Table of Contents

BLESSING	5
PRAYER	6
PREFACE	9
INTRODUCTION	12
Guru Puja Honoring	13
Triphala Eyewash	14
Datun Dant Manjan Oral Hygiene	16
Welcome chant for Belongingness	17
Eyedrops for Lubrication and Cleansing	18
Sun Exercises	19
Asana for Vision	22
Pranayama for Vision	25
Overall Fitness Stretches	26
Snellen Eye Chart	28
Tumbling E Chart	30
Nutrition Watch	32
Tennis Ball Bouncing	34
Skipping	35
Acupressure Walk	36
Meditation	37
Senses are interconnected	38
Aroma for improved Smell	39
Applying Sandal paste	40
Moon and Stars Gazing	41
Participant's Random Act of Kindness	42
Participant's Sankalpa for Eyecare	43
Coconut Oil Eye Massage	44
Acupressure and Reflexology for Eye	45
Marma Points Stimulation	46
Candle Light Trataka	48

    Pinhole Text Reading 50
    Steaming with Eucalyptus Oil 52
    Rosewater Eye Relaxation 53
    Yoganidra 54
    Ashram Experience 55
    Workshops Facilitated 56
    Known Benefits of Workshop 57

PARTING GET TOGETHER 58

GOLDEN RULE 59

PROCESS SEQUENCING 60

PROCESS REGULARITY 60

LIST OF ITEMS 61

ALPHABETICAL LIST OF TERMS 62

REFERENCES 63

EPILOGUE 64

Preface

Eyes are precious. Eyes are the window to the Soul. Healthy eyes reflect Inner peace and radiate Joy. A beautiful face is desired by all, happy Eyes are the key.

Handsome boys and Pretty girls flaunt scintillating eyes.

The Eye Care program is a complete workshop for children, teens and adults to improve vision. Vision is not only physical; it is also about how we perceive the world around us.

Vision includes Day vision, Night vision, Color/Grayscale vision, Peripheral vision.

Far and Near focus must be sharp and eyes must not feel any strain. Eyes should generate proper teardrops and innocently mirror heart's emotions. There should be negligible black spots or webs felt when eyes are shut. There should be good hand-eye coordination.

All are attended to in this program.

Improves immunity and ability to drive confidently at night, read messages with clarity on smart phone, and work on laptop without strain.

Greatly enhances the ability to display and perceive emotions, and infuse life with HAPPINESS.

Did you know that the EYE is the most important sensory organ? The lion's share of our world is transacted through the eyes. All we do or wish to do is first cognized in the Eye.

We express our emotions through the eyes, we speak through the eyes, and we go within with our eyes closed.

ANGER

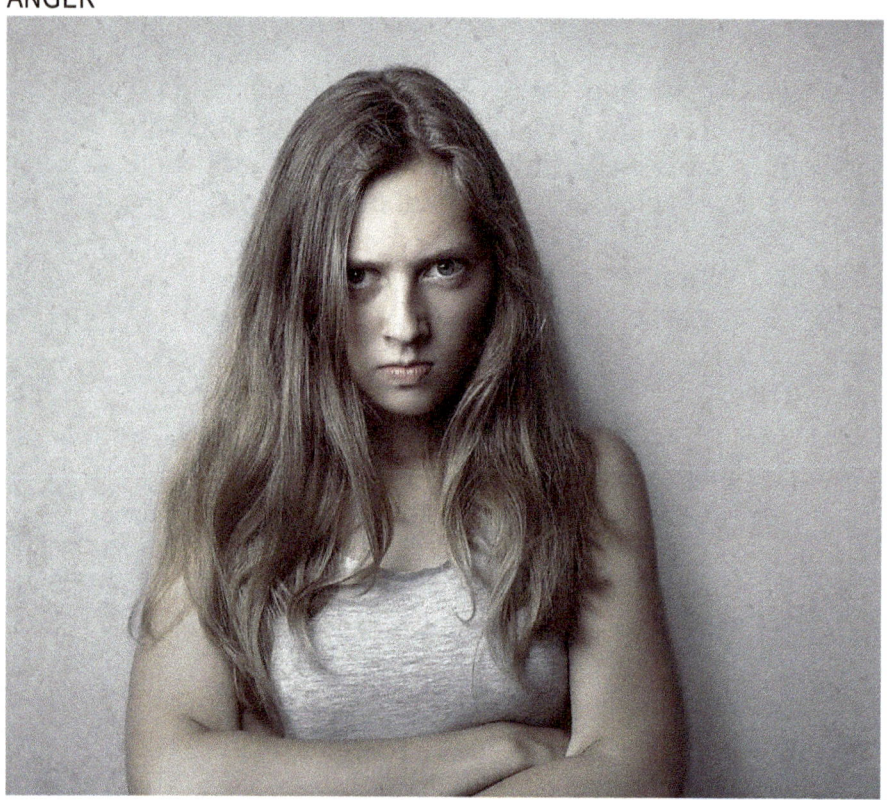

HESITANT   HOPEFUL

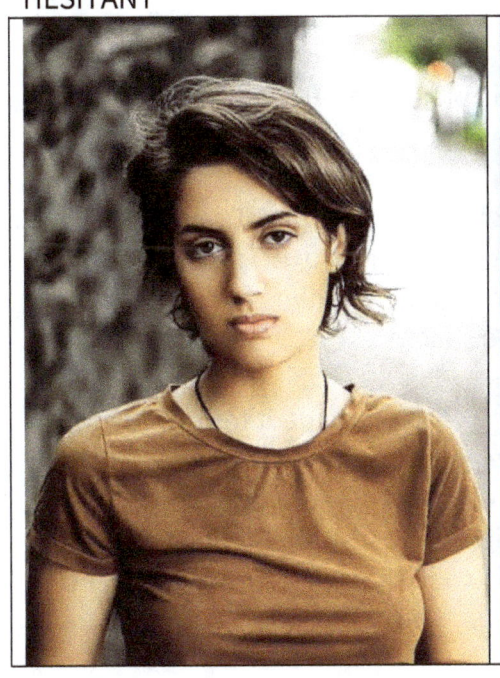
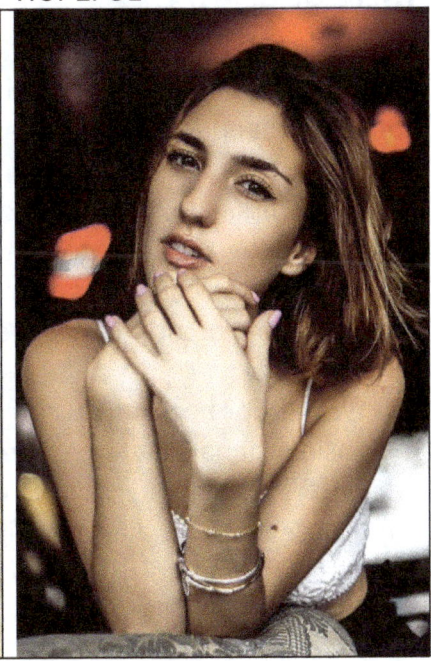

INNOCENCE   JOY

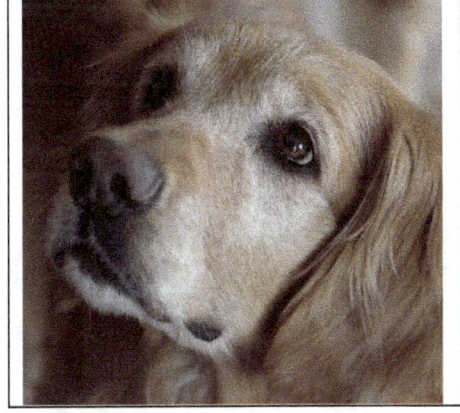
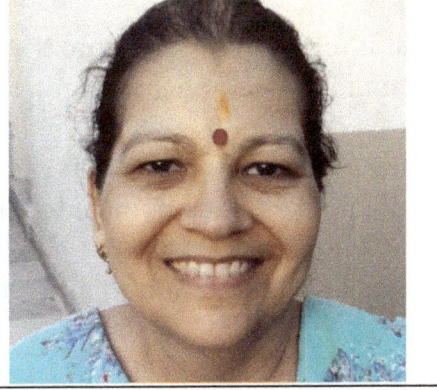

Introduction

A group workshop to improve vision in a carefree, cheerful and collective manner works wonders for all age groups.

A typical workshop consists of 2 hours@day over 10 days. It makes sense if families participate, so that we proactively assist each other during the course, as each aura strengthens the collective forces that make the workshop a success.

Our workshops begin with asking each participant to wash their eyes using triphala water. As the participants come in, the facilitators provide them with freshly prepared triphala water in eye cups. Note that triphala will stain the clothes and washbasin, and we need to be careful. It helps if we do this process in a field or in the open.

Then we move onto oral hygiene, since innumerable studies show that good eyesight is greatly dependent on strong teeth and gums.

This is followed by going into the hall and doing a welcome group chant for moving ahead together in belongingness and confidence.

Many processes make up this wonderful course, there is Yoga and Meditation and Games included. The ending is with a Sankalpa by each participant that shows his commitment towards responsibility for his own fitness, and a group prasadam with havan and singing.

Guru Puja Honoring

Traditionally we perform a guru puja at the course venue. It is to honor the Master whose grace makes it all possible, and to remember the lineage of ancestors who walked this planet, boldly and bravely establishing new ideas, and laying the foundation for respectable and proactive living for generations to come.

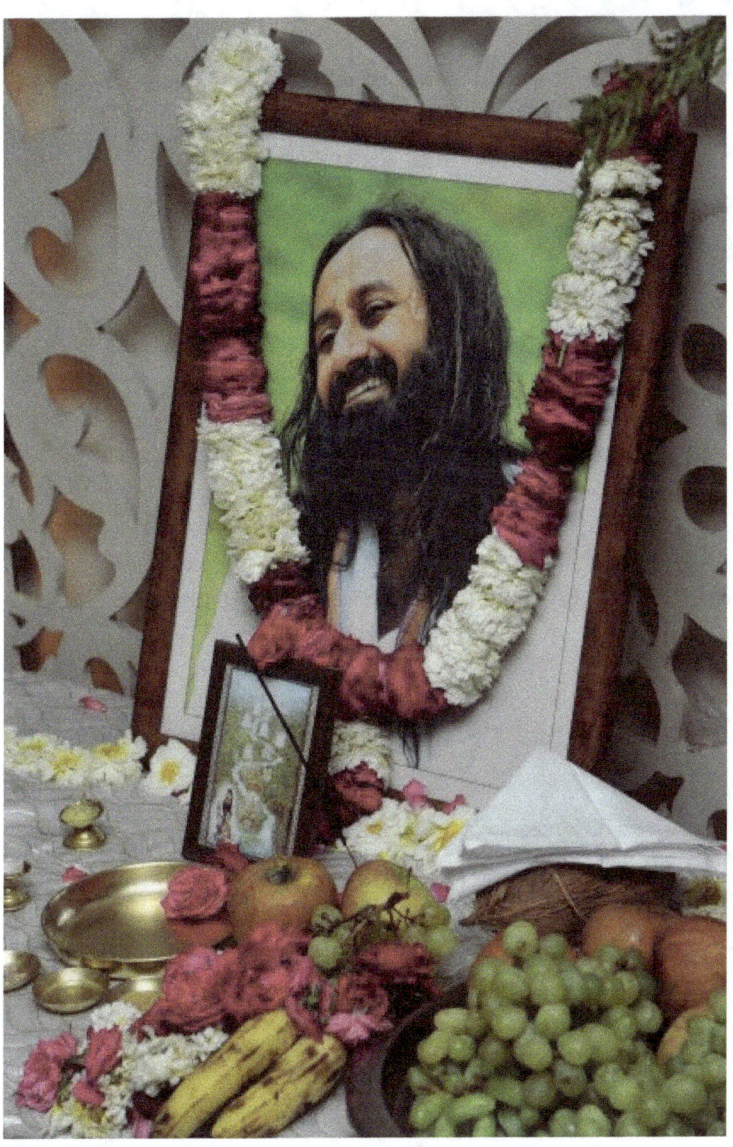

Triphala Eyewash

Triphala churna consists of equal parts of Haritaki (harad or brown myrobalan), Baheda (beleric myrobalan), Amla (Indian gooseberry)

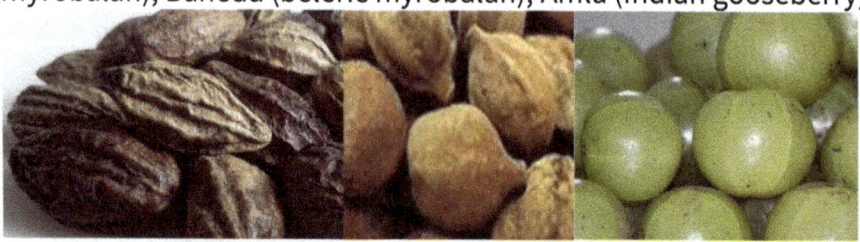

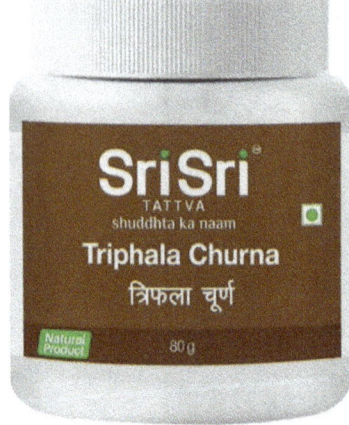

Mix a tablespoon of triphala powder in a liter of water, strain the liquid with fine cloth, and store it in a proper stainless-steel vessel. This triphala water is then used to wash the eyes.

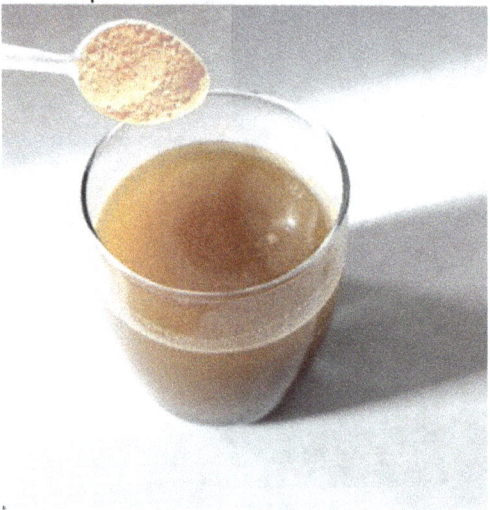

Our program begins with Triphala Eye Wash

This is the first step that we do.

We typically pour the eyewash in an eyecup and dip the eye, and blink a few times. Do with other eye. Repeat by refilling the triphala water a couple of times for both eyes. Finally rinse the eyes with plain water.

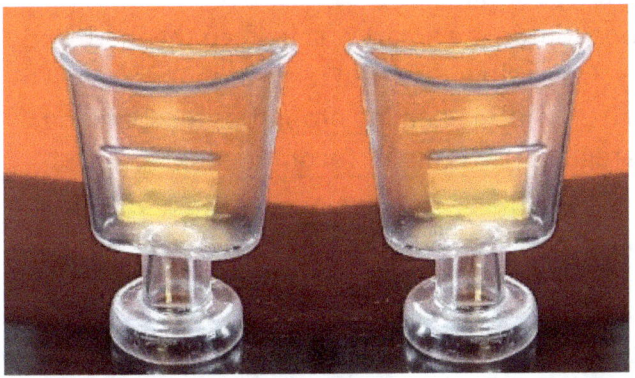

Since triphala water shall stain the surroundings or clothes where it falls, be careful while washing the eyes. In our workshops we prefer to do this process in an open field. At home we can easily do it in our bathroom. It is best to make the water fresh every day.

Sip water after the eyewash.

Datun Dant Manjan Oral Hygiene

It is a sensible practice to have good dental hygiene, since that directly impacts eyesight. Healthy teeth and gums ensure that we shall have good vision.

- Fill the mouth with water, then take water in palm and squirt on forehead thrice
- Put finger on tongue and cough so that we release chest congestion and eye strain
- Neem or Babool datun is a smart way to keep the teeth and gums healthy. Chew slowly with all teeth in sequence.
- Dant Manjan has amazing healing properties for sparkling teeth and its regular use is highly recommended.

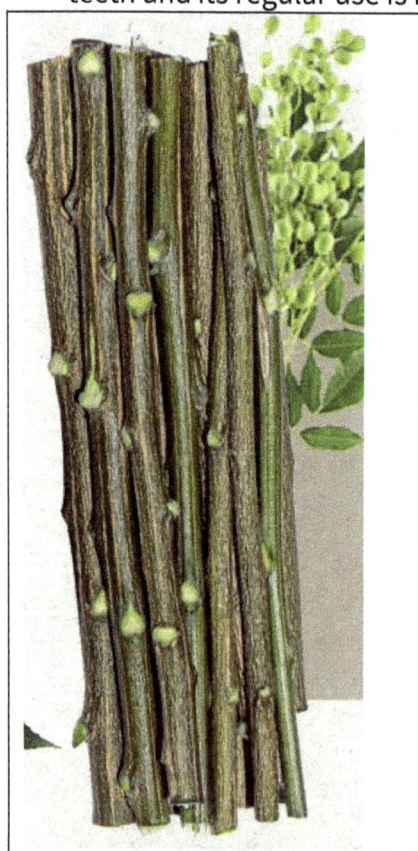
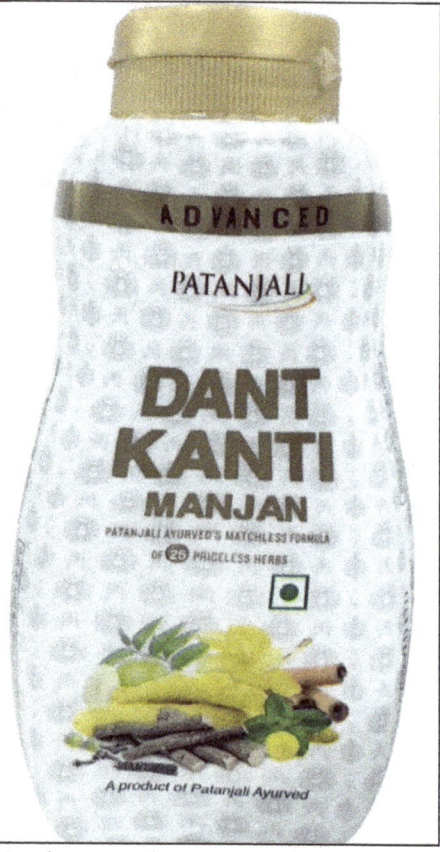

A fluoride free, SLS free toothpaste is also good.
https://www.amazon.in/Bentodent-Organization-Cardamom-Toothpaste-Flouride/dp/B07D7ZFRQ8/

Welcome chant for Belongingness

After the initial processes of eyewash and mouthwash, each participant moves inside the hall. Wipes himself clean with tissues and sits on his Yoga mat.

We begin with a feeling of belongingness – sangat chatwam.
- Inhale deeply a few times, and chant Om together.
- Recite a verse from the Bhagavad Gita.

सर्वधर्मान् परित्यज्य , माम् एकं शरणं व्रज ।

अहं त्वा सर्वपापेभ्यः , मोक्षयिष्यामि मा शुचः ॥ 18.66

sarvadharmān parityajya , mām ekaṃ śaraṇaṃ vraja |
ahaṃ tvā sarvapāpebhyaḥ , mokṣayiṣyāmi mā śucaḥ || 18.66
<u>Meaning</u>
Follow me completely with intense faith and know with conviction that you are taken care of, you are healed and whole, no fear.

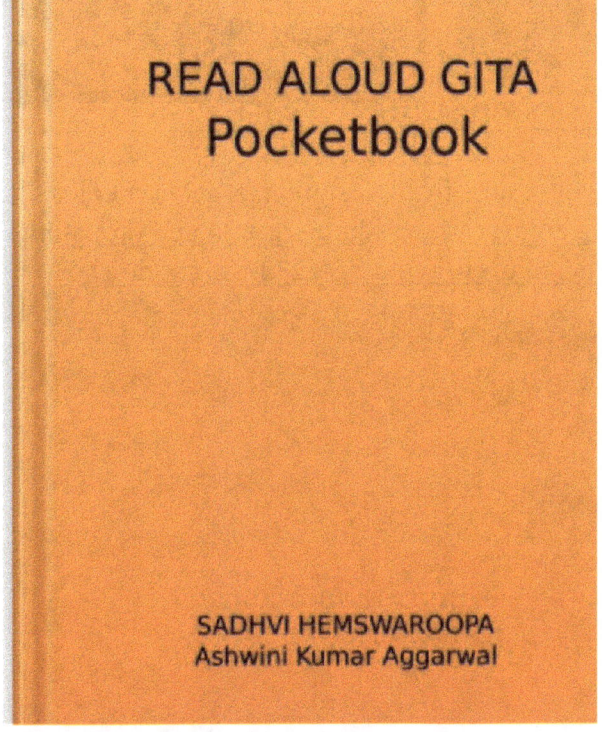

Eyedrops for Lubrication and Cleansing

- It is essential to keep the eyes clean and well lubricated. Using good quality herbal eyedrops is recommended.
- Lie down on the yoga mat and carefully put eyedrops. Blink a few times, then get up and go outside to the fresh air and sunlight for sun exercises.

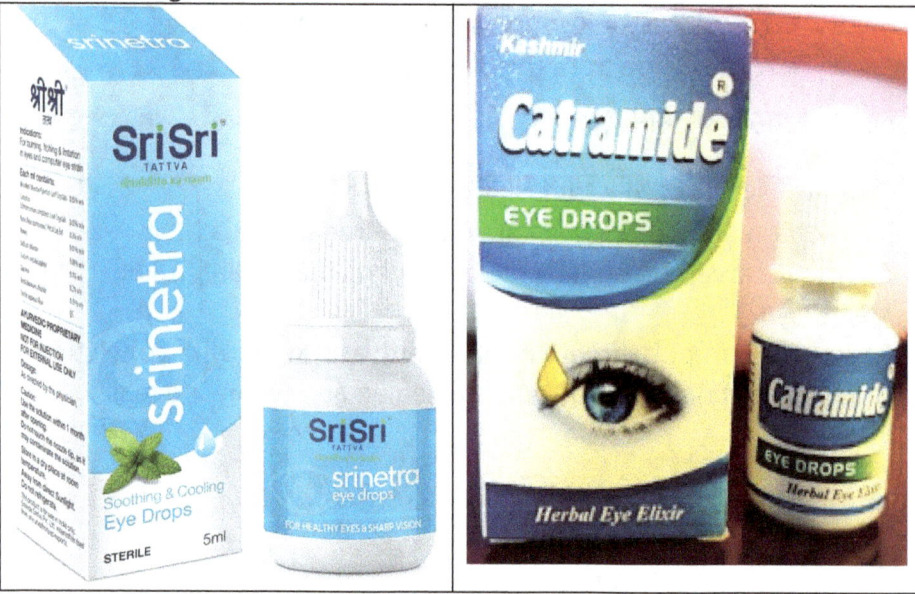

We may use Catramide eyedrops from Kashmir Herbal Remedies.
https://www.srisritattva.com/products/shop-srinetra-eye-drops-5ml
https://ayurcentralonline.com/en/eye-care/2283-catramide-eye-drops-10ml.html

Sun Exercises

First we put eyedrops, then we move to the sunlight.

We spend 20 minutes doing eye movements in sunlight. These are:
- **Facing the dawn sun** or at dusk, close the eyes, so that the sunlight falls on the closed eyelids and you feel the light sensation. Keeping the eyes closed, move the head slowly left to right.

Now open the eyes and turn your back to the sun.

- **Left to Right** slow stepwise eye movement, with normal blinking, focusing at each step for a second.
- **Top to Bottom** eye switching – hold gaze towards top for 5 seconds, lower gaze for 1 second, back and forth.
- **Far and Near** object focus – focus on the farthest object you can clearly see, hold for few seconds, then switch gaze to the nearest object you can clearly see.
- **Double Blur** – extend your fingers wide and look through them to far, then bring the gaze back to look at the finger.

Each sun exercise is to be done for few minutes duration.

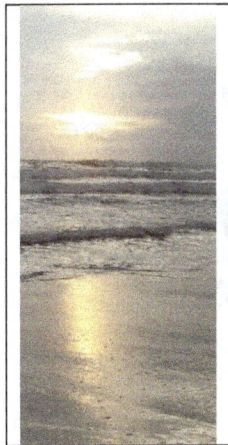
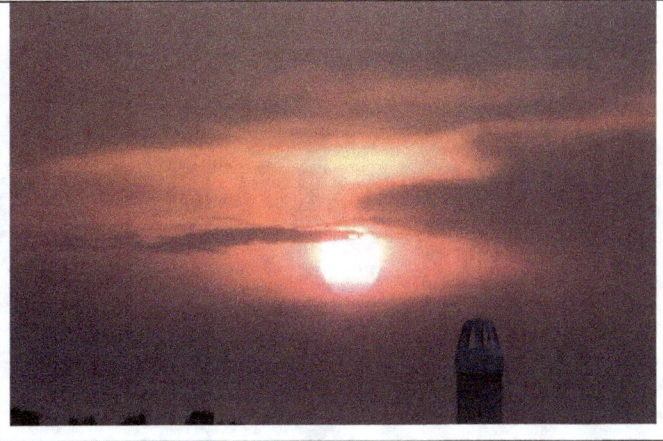

Sip water after the Sunning.

FACING the SUN with CLOSED EYES and HEAD Movements

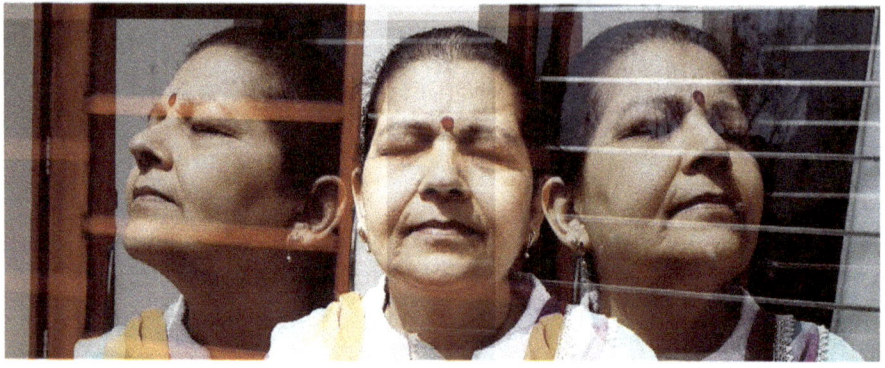

Head Still, Eyes LEFT to RIGHT and RIGHT to LEFT

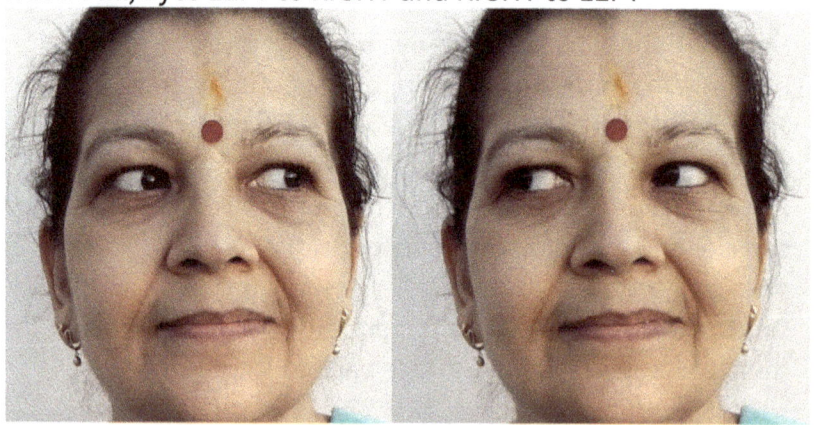

Head Still, Eyes TOP to BOTTOM and BOTTOM to TOP

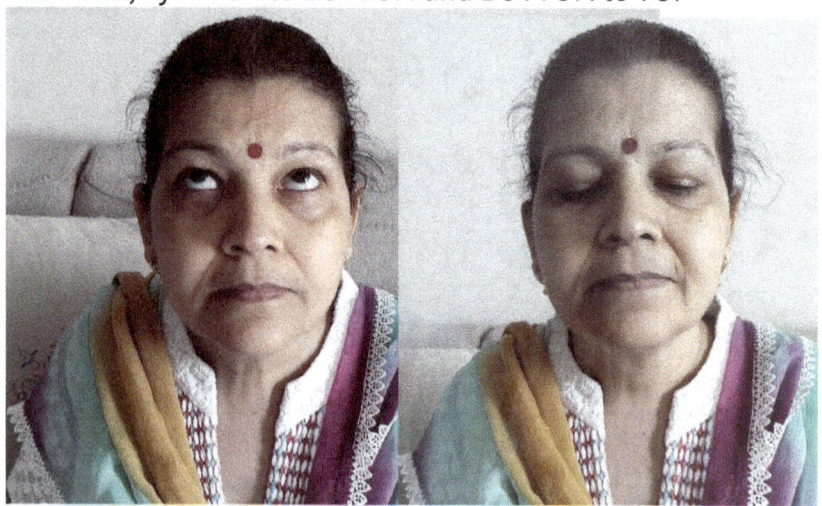

FAR and NEAR

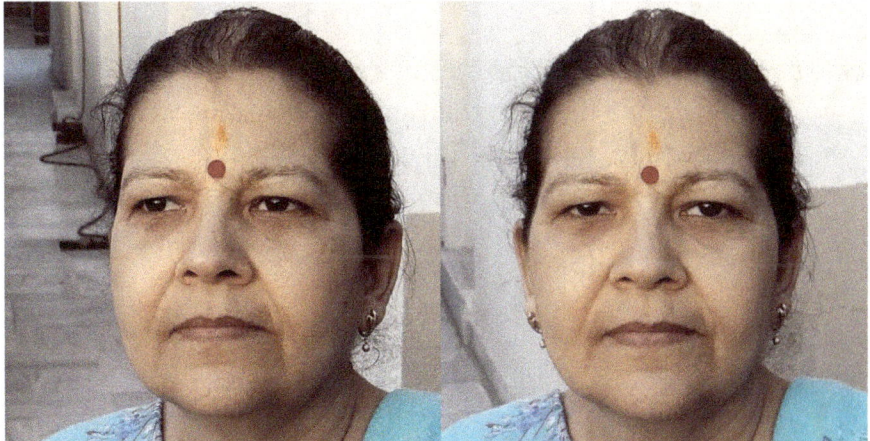

DOUBLE BLUR

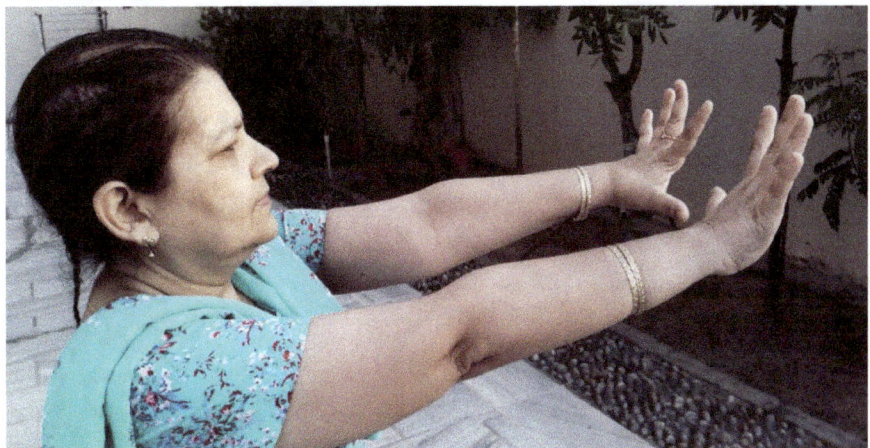

Extend the hands with fingers wide. Look through gap between the fingers to any far object. Hold gaze for few moments. Then bring back gaze to look at a finger. Hold gaze for a few moments. Repeat. You may notice a blurring or a double vision of the fingers.

Note: Some days it will be cloudy or raining. So we do the sun exercises in the hall using a high wattage incandescent lamp.
https://www.amazon.in/Philips-BR125-Light-Bulb-250/dp/B002B522SU/

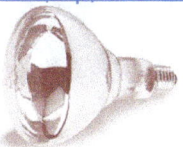

Asana for Vision

Come back from the sunlight to do some stretches.
- Bhujangasana to strengthen spine and flex the whole body
- Naukasana to hold eyes, fingers, toes steady
- Simhasana to open the larynx and tone throat and eyes

BHUJANGASANA - COBRA

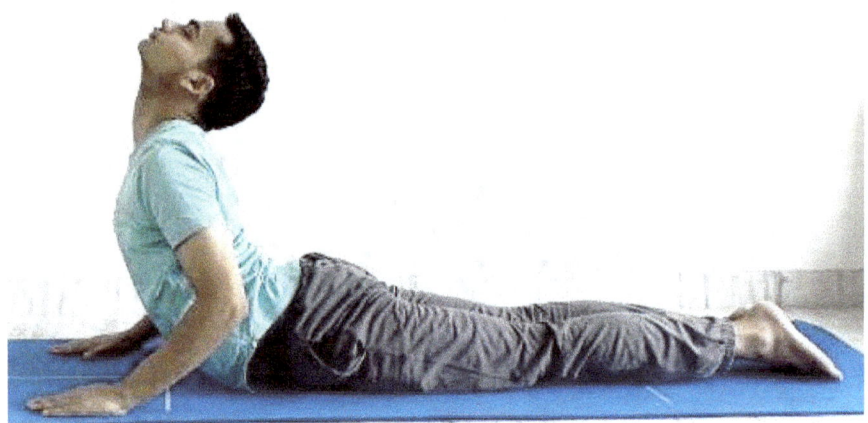

NAUKASANA – BOAT

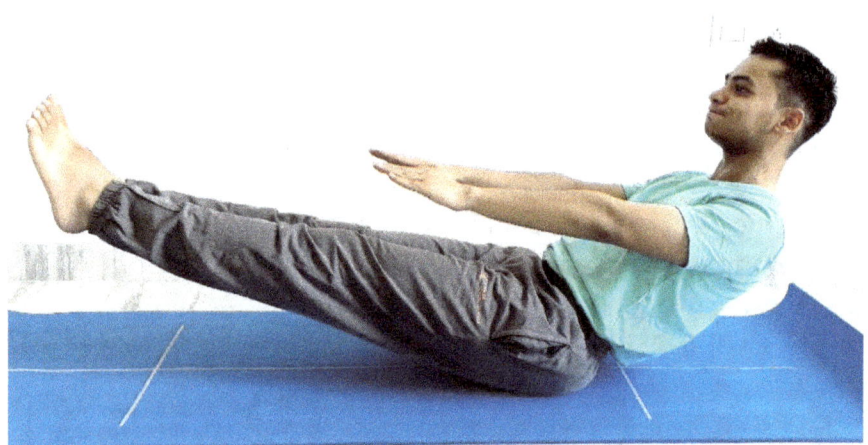

SIMHASANA – LION	SARVANGASANA – Shoulder Stand
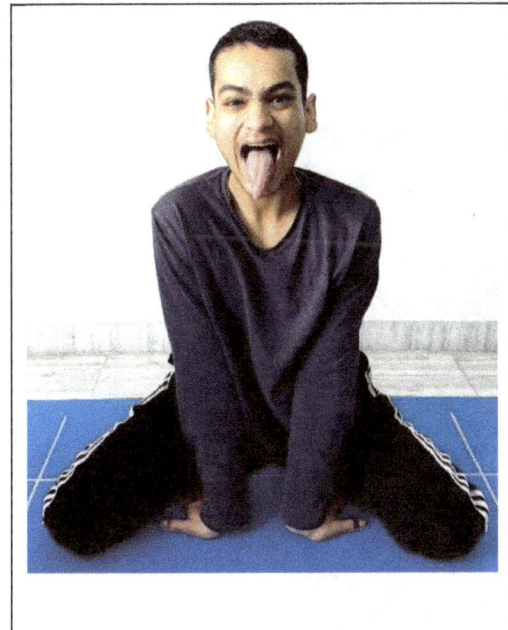	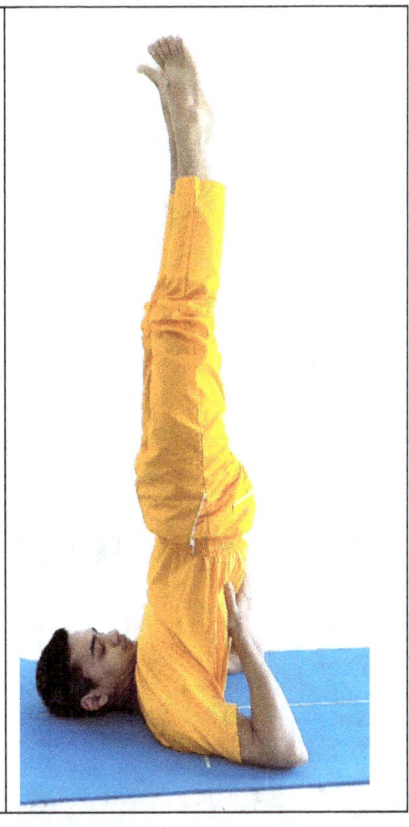

EYE MOVEMENTS

- Fast blinking so the eyes feel thoroughly energized. Follow it up with tightly Squeezing shut and Opening thrice. Then do hot palming thrice
- Clockwise and anticlockwise eye movements
- Diagonal eye movements

FAST BLINKING – OPEN and CLOSE the EYES rapidly

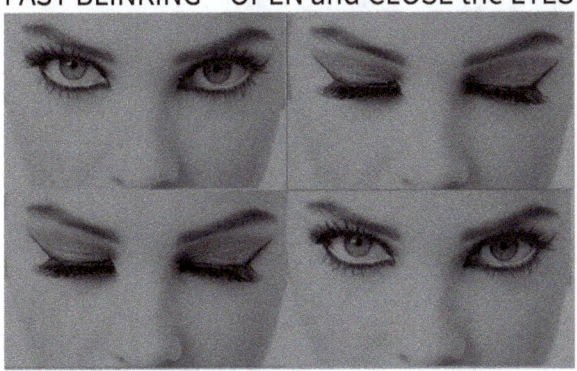

EYE ROTATION – Keep the head steady with hand support. Move the eyeball slowly in a circle. First clockwise then anticlockwise. Then look at the ceiling diagonally upwards and then downwards to the floor. Repeat in alternate direction.

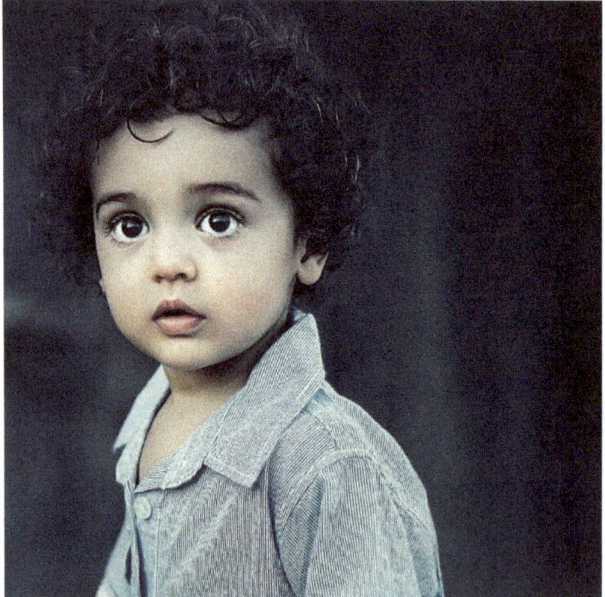

EYE SQUEEZE

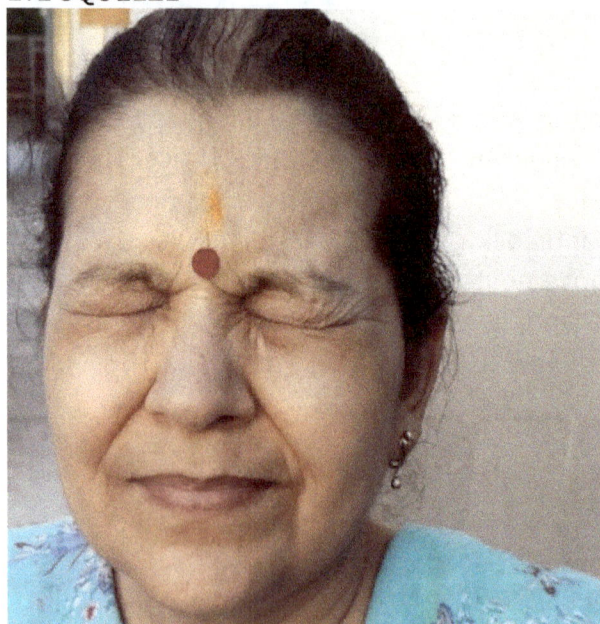

Each exercise is for a minute or two.

Pranayama for Vision

Sit straight with spine erect and relaxed shoulders. Take slow deep breaths.

Now do Mudra Pranayama.
- Hands in **Prana Mudra** and do deep breathing. In this mudra we keep the Index and Middle fingers straight, and the ring finger and little finger touch the tip of thumb.
- Hands in **Vayu Mudra** and do deep breathing. In this mudra we touch the index finger to the base of the thumb. Rest three fingers are straight.

Each mudra is for a couple of minutes.

PRANA MUDRA – Index finger and Middle finger straight, ring finger and little finger touching the thumb (left image).

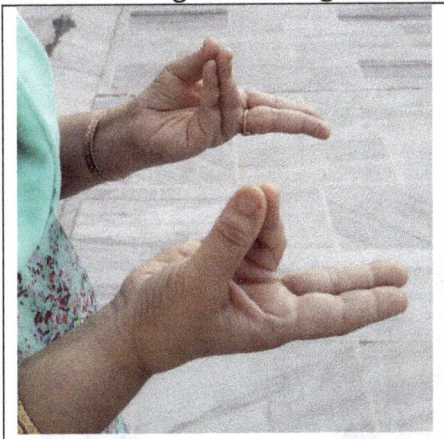
PRANA Mudra

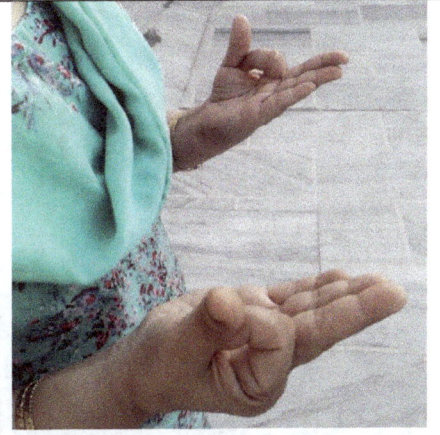
VAYU Mudra

VAYU MUDRA – Index finger touching base of thumb, rest three fingers straight (right image).

We may also do **Khechari Mudra**. Curl the tongue backwards in the mouth and rub the depression in the soft palate with the tip of the tongue for a few seconds.

Take a Sip of water.

Overall Fitness Stretches

- Superbrain Yoga
- Butterfly
- Spine slide
- Extend hands to side, with outstretched palms do bye bye
- Stretch arms in front, extended fingers, pull back from wrist
- Neck and Shoulder movements

Stretches that improve digestion ultimately impact the eyes favorably as well.

TITLI ASANA – BUTTERFLY

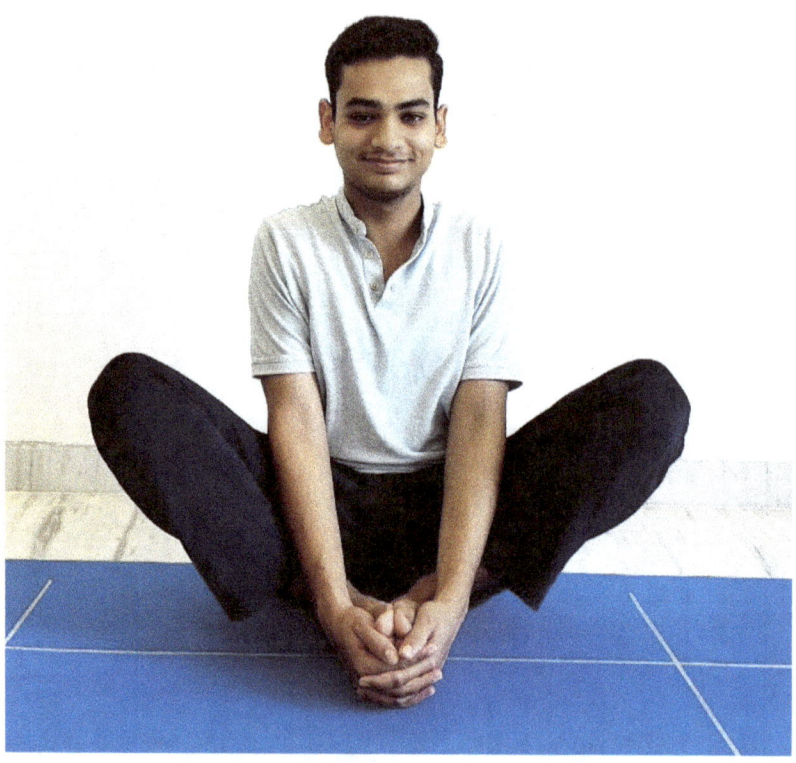

Now that we are all wide awake and alert, we can do a self visual acuity test using EYE CHARTS.

When
- every breath I breathe
- each step I take
- the faintest move I make

is directly willed by my Lord Sri Krishna

I have the faith I can make myself strong, humble and pleasant. This is also what this workshop hopes to achieve.

A HAPPY GROUP AFTER A RELAXING WORKSHOP SESSION

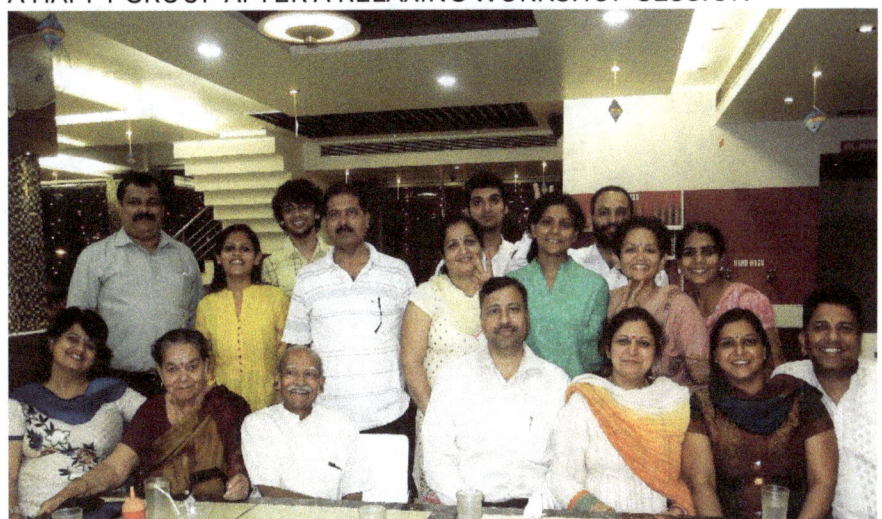

The Snellen Chart named after its founder is written here in font **Carlito**, a sans serif font. It is also seen in font **Rockwell** which is a serif font.

This chart is commonly used for Visual Acuity Testing.

Snellen Eye Chart

E	1	20/200
F P	2	20/100
T O Z	3	20/70
L P E D	4	20/50
P E C F D	5	20/40
E D F C Z P	6	20/30
F E L O P Z D	7	20/25
D E F P O T E C	8	20/20
L E F O D P C T	9	20/15
F D P L T C E O	10	20/13
P E Z O L C F T D	11	20/10

Vision testing uses the Snellen Eye chart, which requires a test distance of 20 feet. Printout in high resolution on A3 size paper.

During the eye test, be 20 feet from the Snellen Chart, under good lighting conditions.

Cover your right eye and read the chart using the left eye starting at the top and proceeding downwards until you can't distinguish the letters.

Then switch the eyes and repeat the process from the same viewing distance.

The line with the smallest visible letter size gives your results for each eye.

NORMAL VISION is called 6/6 or 20/20
The first number in the fraction refers to your testing distance in feet, and the second number refers to the distance in feet someone with "normal" vision can clearly see.

E.g., 20/20 vision means that you can see an object from 20 feet.
E.g., 20/30 vision means that you can see an object from 20 feet which ideally can be seen from 30 feet.

20 feet is equivalent to 6.096 meters; hence 20/20 vision is equal to 6/6 vision in metric system.

NOTE on Vision 20/10
It is seen that some people have excellent vision, so the category 20/10 is also there. It means that what a person can normally see from 10 feet, is clearly visible to the exceptional eyesight from a distance of 20 feet! Such vision is much sought for in aeronautics and space careers.

Tumbling E Chart

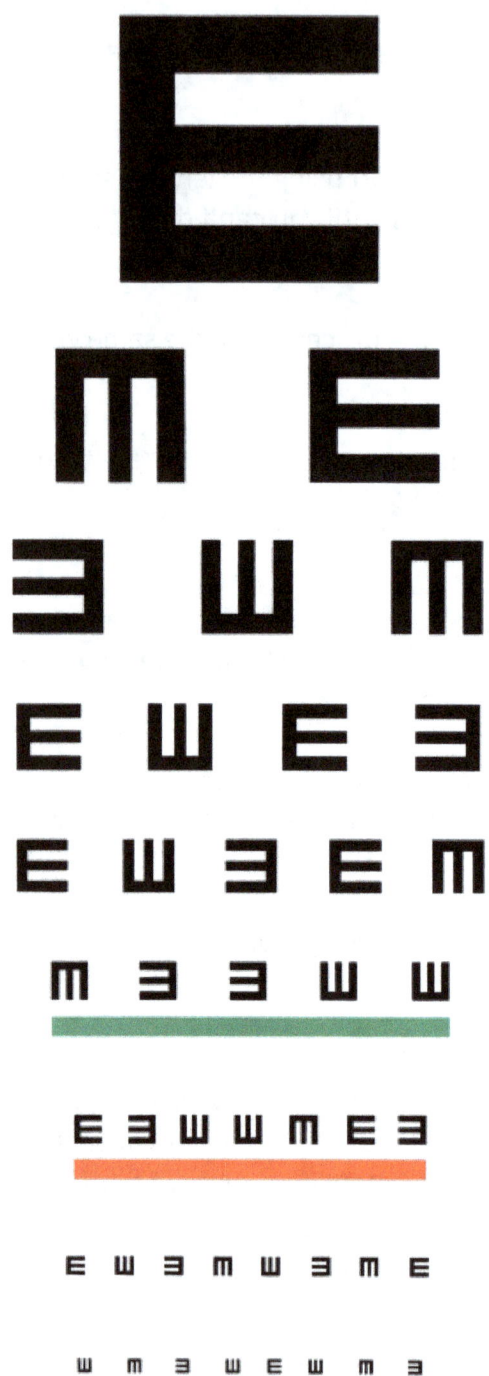

Vision testing also uses the Tumbling E chart, which requires a test distance of 10 feet. Printout in high resolution on A3 size paper.

1. Place the chart on a wall at a distance of 10 feet.
2. Cover one eye completely.
3. Start with the first line at the top of the chart and point with your fingers the direction the "fingers" on the E are pointing.
4. Point to each "E" going left to right from top to bottom.
5. When you fail to correctly identify the orientation of at least 50 percent of the Es on a line, stop the test and note the previous line you were able to correctly identify at least 50% of the tumbling E's.
6. Repeat the above steps for the other eye.

After the self-checkup, we honor ourselves with something to eat. Preferably some almonds soaked overnight and a glass of fresh juice or milk.

Nutrition Watch

Proper nutrition helps a lot in good eyesight. One must have fresh vegetables and fruits in the diet regularly.

- Slowly chew 3 almonds soaked overnight.

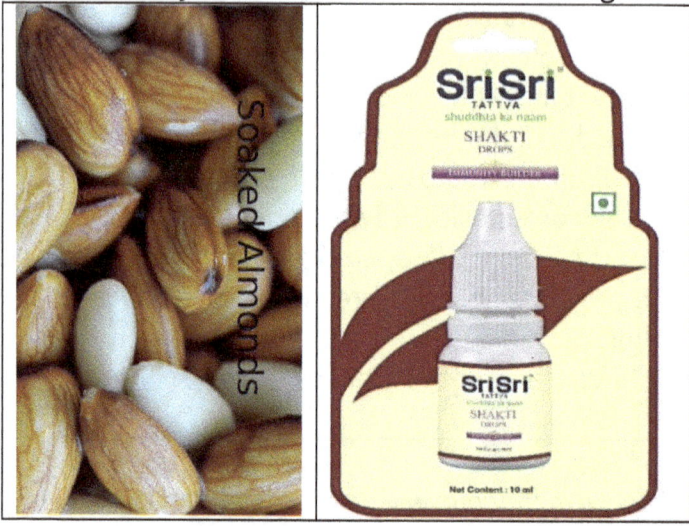

- Drink a glass of carrot juice, containing carrots, celery (ajmoda leaves), lemon (or orange), ginger, mint (pudina).

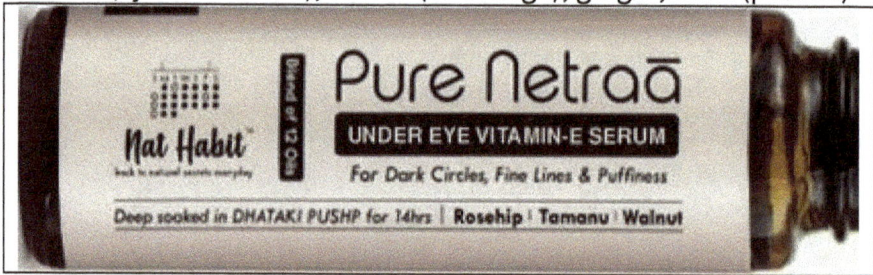

- Shakti drops drink with water regularly.
- Vitamin E serum apply under the eyes.

https://nathabit.in/collections/pure-netraa

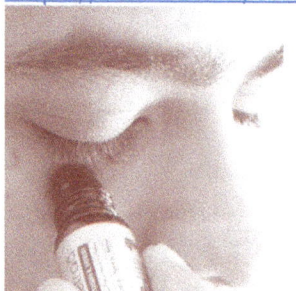

FOODS for EYE HEALTH

Nutrient	Source
Vitamin A	Apricot, Carrot, Mango, Sweet potato, Spinach
Vitamin C	Amla, Broccoli, Orange
Vitamin E	Almond, Spinach, Wheat germ
Omega 3 fatty acids	Flaxseed, Walnut
Lutein	Orange, Papaya, Lettuce

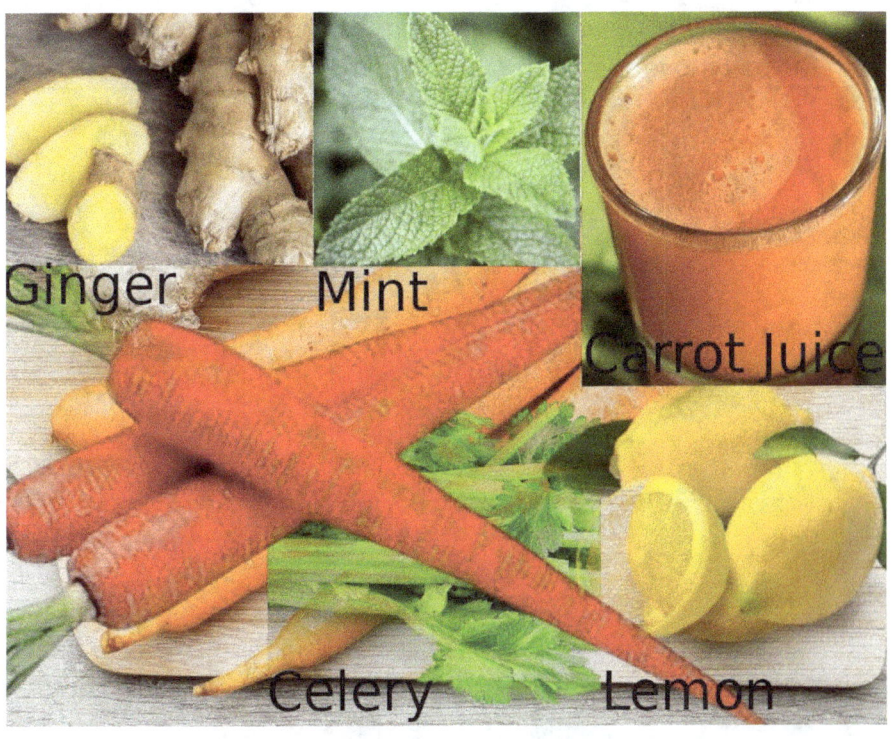

After food, we are ready for a game. Distribute the tennis balls and all begin to play. If you are doing it in the hall, stack the Yoga mats and belongings to one side so there is enough space.

Tennis Ball Bouncing

Outdoor games like table tennis, badminton, and lawn tennis are a great means to keep the body fit and the mind flexible. These aid brain-body-eye coordination and help in improving eyesight tremendously. The sport is to be played for 10-15 minutes.

In our workshops we play a game using tennis balls, each participant does his own thing, catching/bowling/bouncing, whatever. The idea is to be alert and keep moving the eyes in sync with the ball movement.

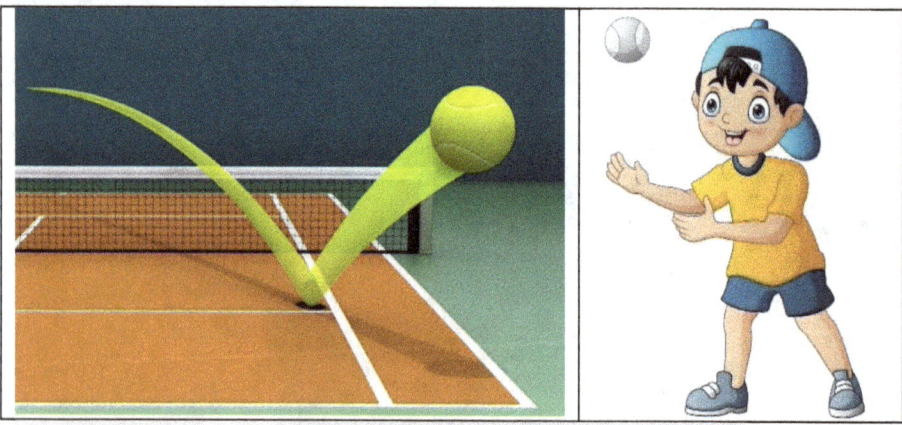

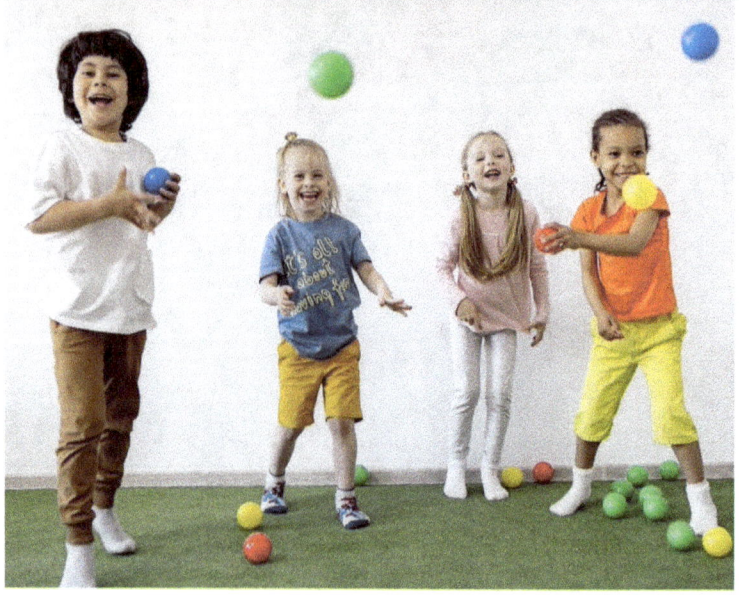

Skipping

Skipping is another great method to improve hand-eye coordination and increase overall fitness. Use a skipping rope as per your height and gaily do 100 skips.

Laugh and talk while skipping and also keep count. Notice if your skipping speed and count increase day by day with regular practice.

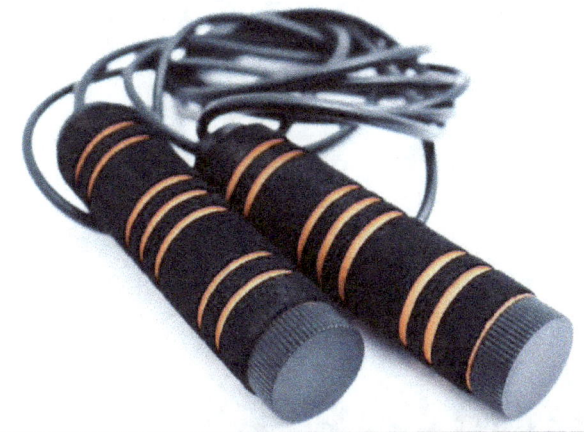

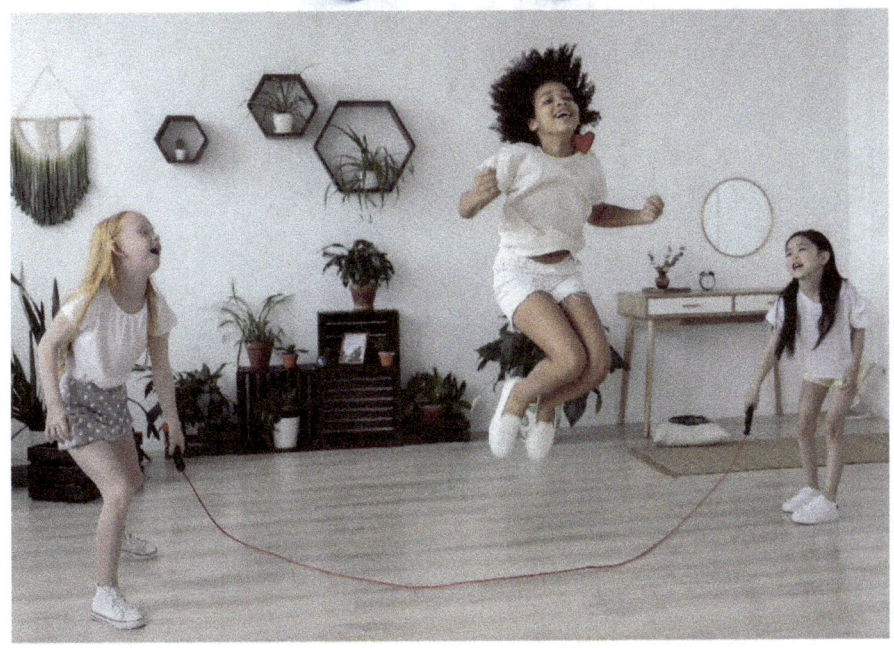

Acupressure Walk

Use an acupressure mat to stimulate the points in the feet. Many parks now have foot reflexology walking tracks, these are beneficial in tackling a variety of blockages in the nervous system, including easing eye afflictions. Even high-quality Reflexology Slippers can work wonders. Walk for 10 minutes on the acupressure.

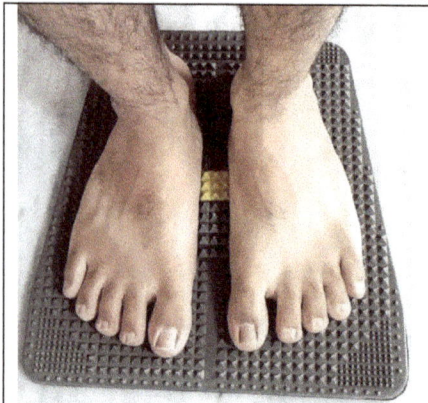
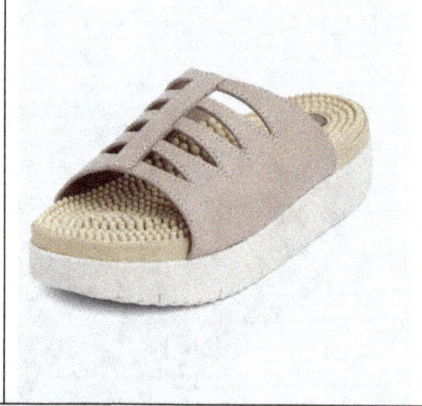

https://kenkoh.jp/in/product/taiyo-nude/

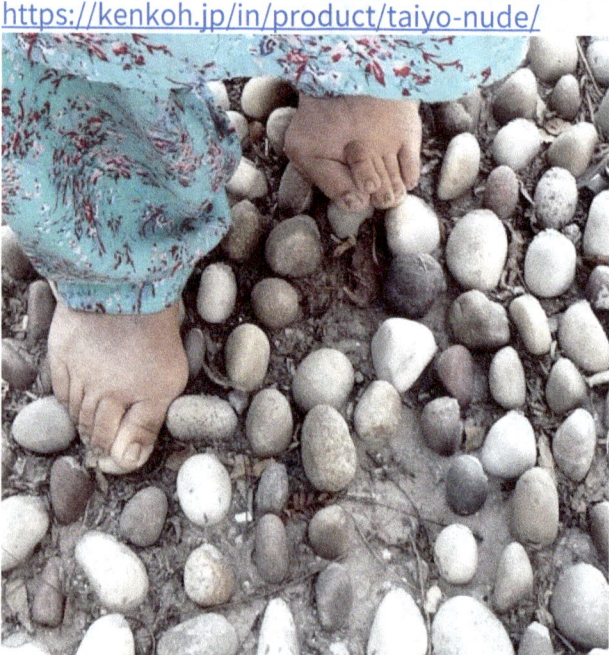

For home use get a high-quality acupressure mat e.g. https://www.akuspike.com/

Meditation

We sit down comfortably on our seats for a guided meditation. It is good to use any meditation from Gurudev's series. E.g., *Healing Through Breath | Day 1 of 10 Days Breath and Meditation Journey with Gurudev*
https://www.youtube.com/watch?v=BKsw1abYwdg

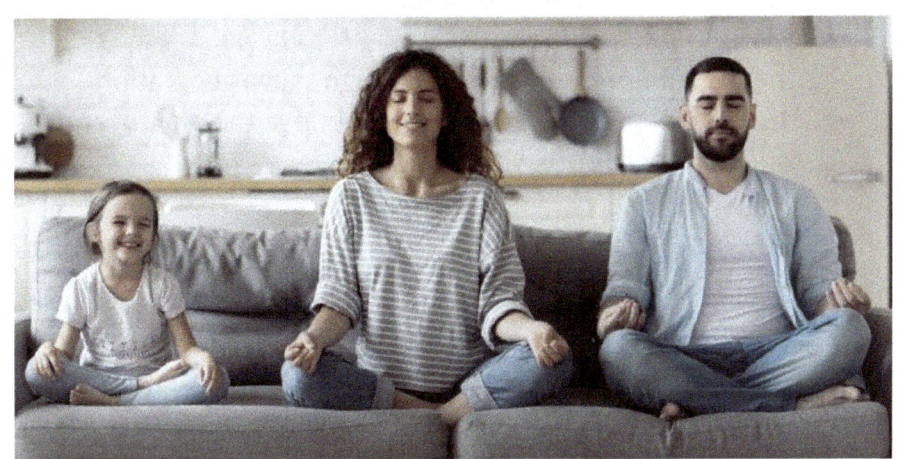

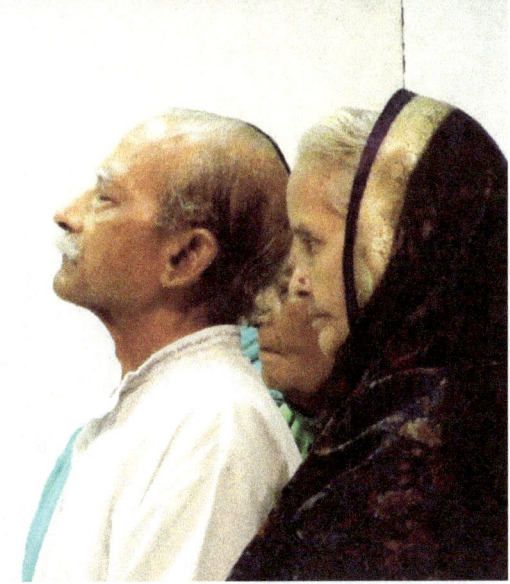

Sip water after Meditation.

Senses are interconnected

When we take good care of one sense faculty, the other senses will naturally get better. Hence in our workshops, we make it a point to ensure oral hygiene, skin tone up, aroma therapy, and sound healing through guided meditation and chanting.

- Chew one Neem Leaf thoroughly with proper saliva generation.
- Chew an Almond slowly with enough saliva generation.
- Sip water very slowly, turning it around in the mouth, and touching each tooth with the tongue.

Aroma for improved Smell

Pass around a basket of fragrant flowers, e.g., jasmine or rose, so that each participant can take a good deep smell.

We can also use an essential oil as diffuser. E.g., lavender or frankincense.
https://phool.co/collections/essential-oils/products/phool-essential-oil-lavender

https://phool.co/collections/essential-oils/products/phool-essential-oil-frankincense

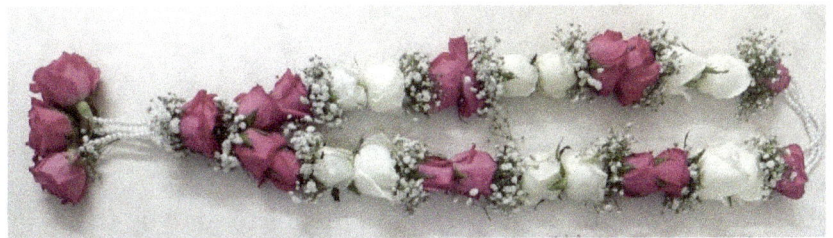

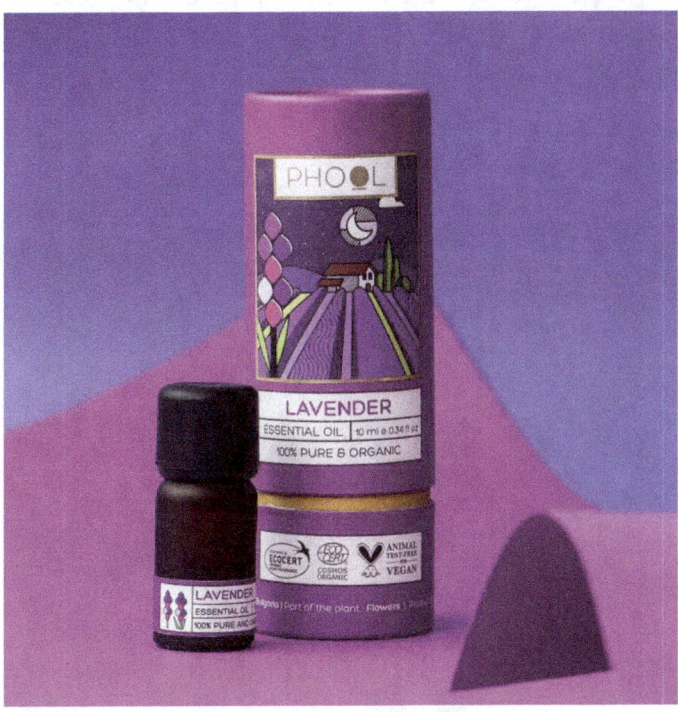

Applying Sandal paste

Spend a few minutes rubbing a sandalwood stick on the wet grinding stone until a thick paste is generated. Apply it on the forehead and on the face. Wipe it clean whenever.

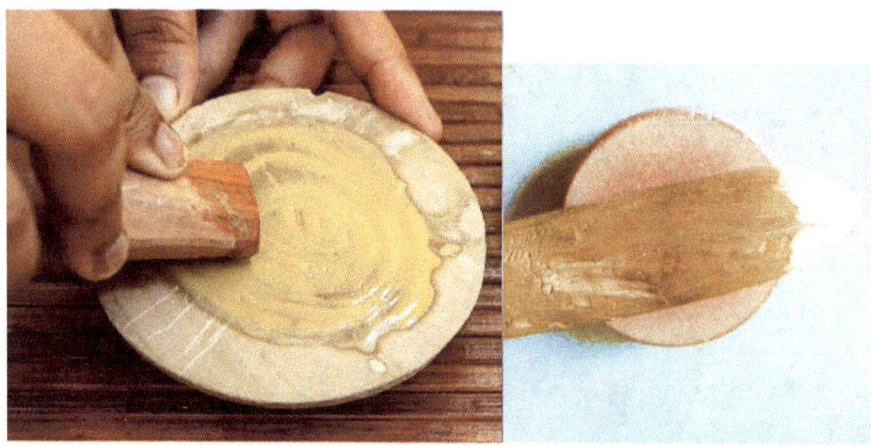

Even the process of rubbing is an intense means to tone up the digestive system and all organs in the abdomen. A proper digestion ensures flawless eyesight.

Moon and Stars Gazing

Though this is not a part of the workshop, but a gentle reminder is given to all that they may spend ten minutes gazing at the stars and the moon during nighttime. The soothing starlight and the moon rays help activate some glands and trigger some enzymes that go a long way in making the eyes happy and sharp.

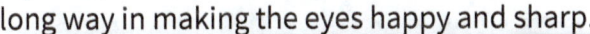

Participant's Random Act of Kindness

It is now time for the participants to make a commitment for society. Ask each participant as to what he shall do during the day that shall bring a smile to someone.

Even the simplest task is welcome, e.g.,
- phoning one's grandparents,
- tidying one's cupboard,
- helping someone less fortunate in anyway.

Pass the mike around as each participant affirms his vision for a better society.

Participant's Sankalpa for Eyecare

A beautiful process is the Sankalpa. Each participant makes a commitment regarding responsibility for his own health, especially eyecare. Pass the mike around and make each one state his wish as to what eyecare habit he shall cultivate.

Even a general task like walking every day or getting up early in the morning is to be appreciated by a round of applause.

Coconut Oil Eye Massage

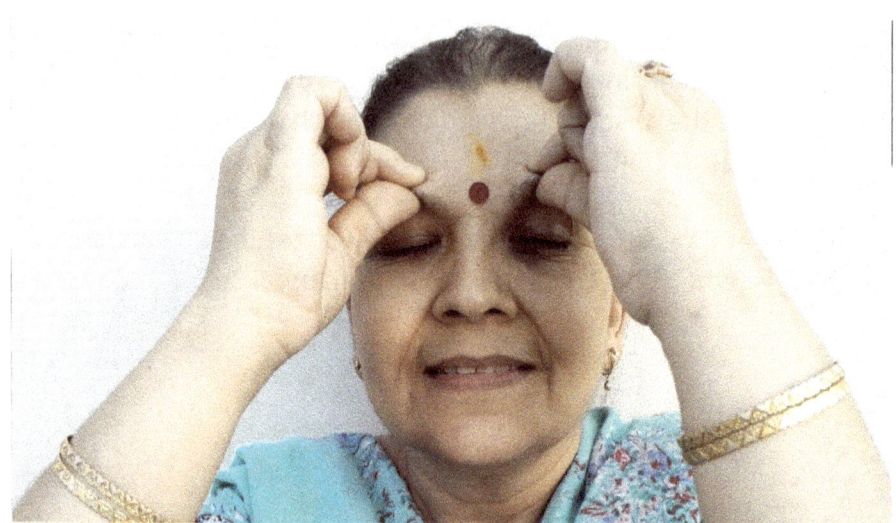

Clean your hands thoroughly. Apply a few drops of oil on the closed eyelids and do gentle massage with finger tips. Slowly press the eye-sockets using thumb and index finger.

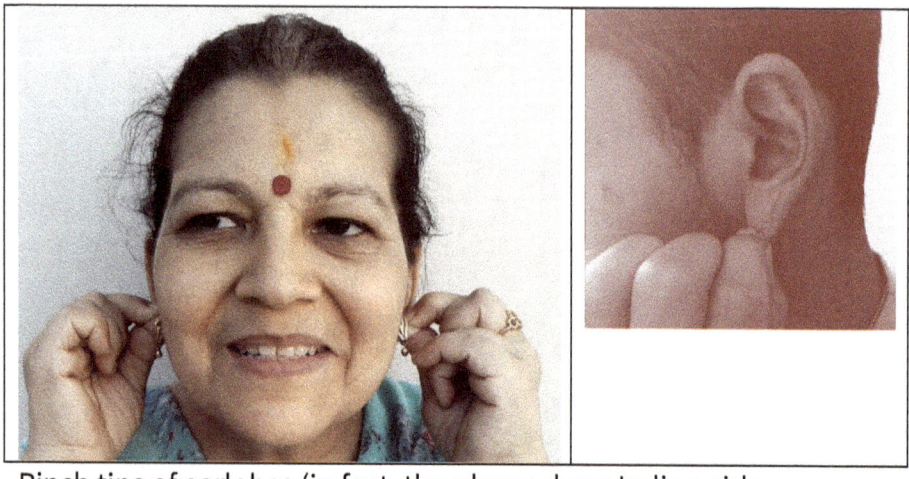

Pinch tips of earlobes (in fact, the place where Indian girls wear earrings is the correct point). Massage the ears and temples thoroughly.

Acupressure and Reflexology for Eye

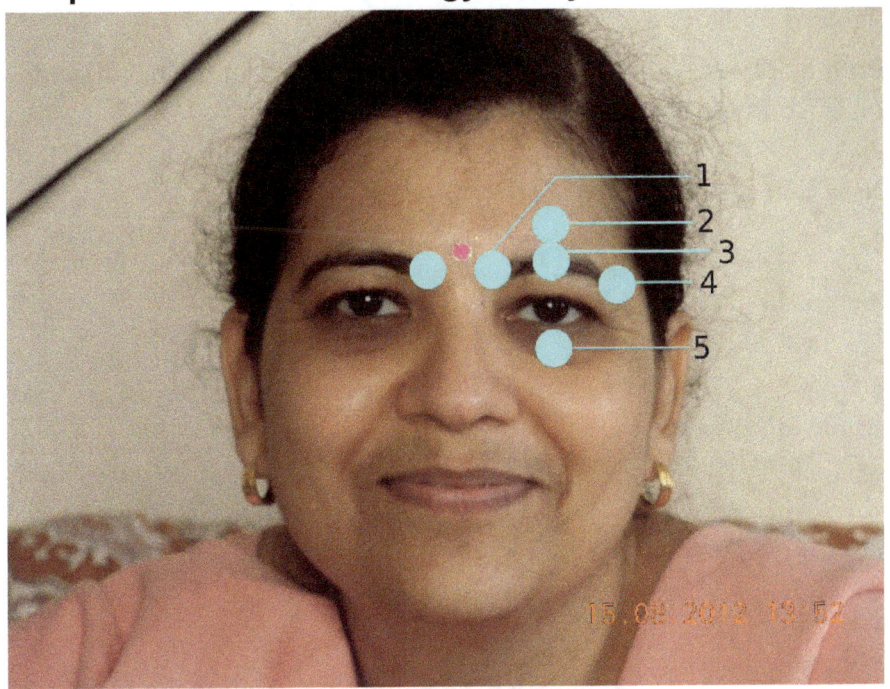

https://joyretcmedispa.com/5-acupressure-points-for-eye-relief/
https://chinesefootreflexology.com/how-to-reverse-age-related-vision-problems-and-start-seeing-clearly-again/

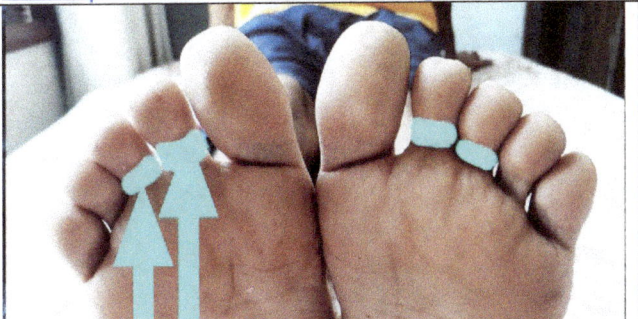 Left Sole = Points for RIGHT Eye Right Sole = Points for LEFT Eye These points are at the joining of the second and third fingers to the foot. Foot acupressure points enhance the eyesight by strengthening eye muscles & correcting refraction to some degree	EyeAcupressure Points Relieve 1.Sinus, Watery 2.Glaucoma, Twitching 3.Redness, Pain 4.Migraine 5.Conjunctivitis, Swelling hence makes eyes very healthy

Marma Points Stimulation

Pour a drop of oil in the nail gap of both big toes, in the navel, and on the bony part behind the ears.

NAIL GAP of BIG TOE

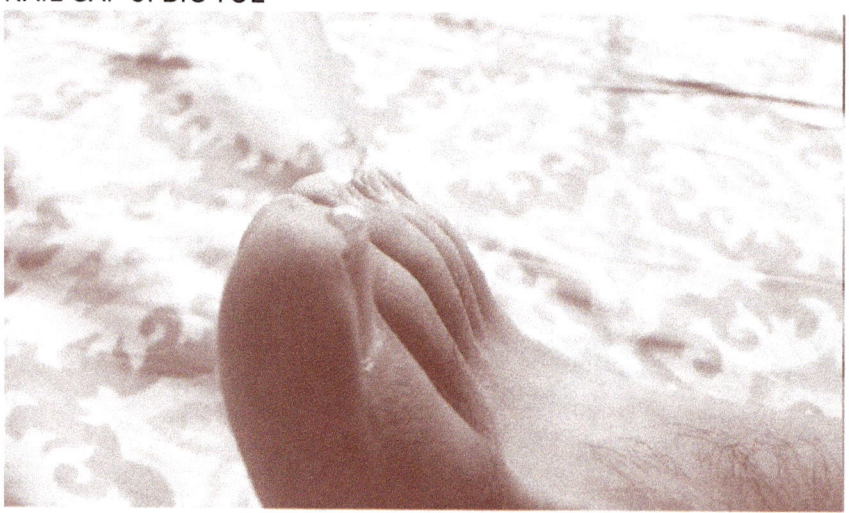

BELLY BUTTON

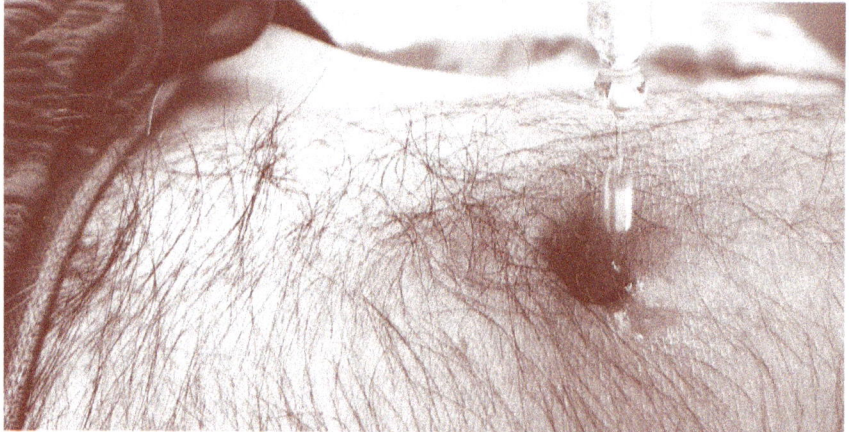

BEHIND the EAR

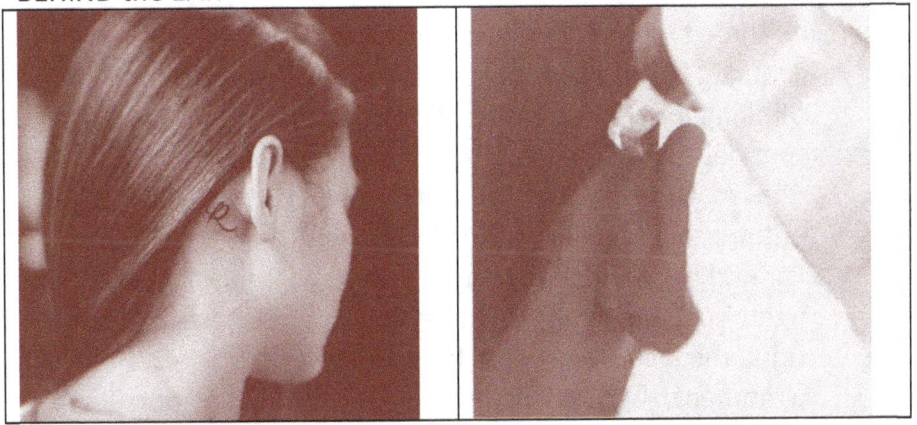

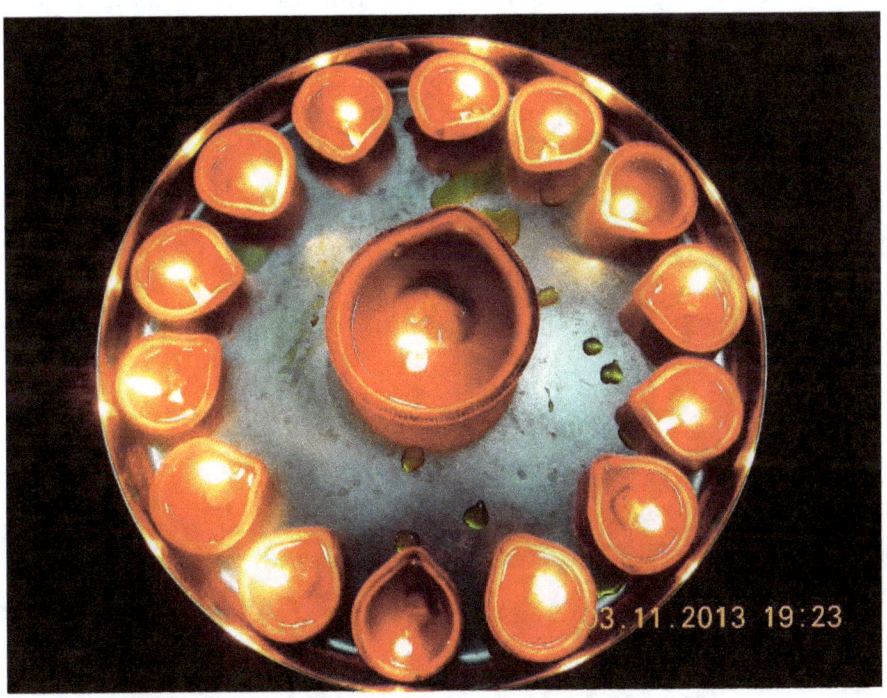

Candle Light or a lighted traditional Diwali Diya is used for improving near vision.

Candle Light Trataka

There are three types of candle light exercises.
- Trataka. In this we gaze at a flicker free flame without blinking for a few minutes till the eyes begin to water. After that palm the eyes for a few minutes. Then lie down in Shavasana using cool rosewater swabs on the eyes. The entire process takes ten to fifteen minutes.
- Far and near body movements sitting in front of candle light. Keep the candle flame at eye level. Sit relaxed. Now bring the face close to the flame up to a few inches. Hold for a moment, then slowly rock back to normal position. Repeat for few minutes. Blink normally.
- Observing colors in the flame. In this process we simply notice the colors we see in the flame. Orange, yellow, grey, blue, or any other color. Just observe closely for a few minutes. Blink normally.

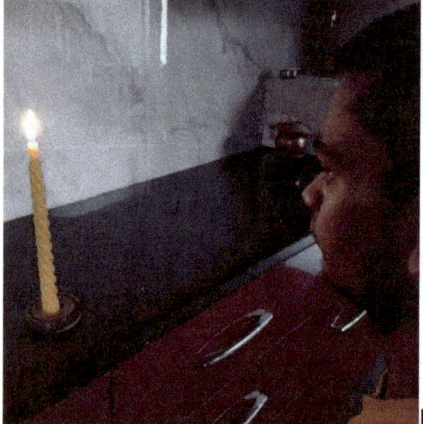
EYES in Line with Tip of Flame

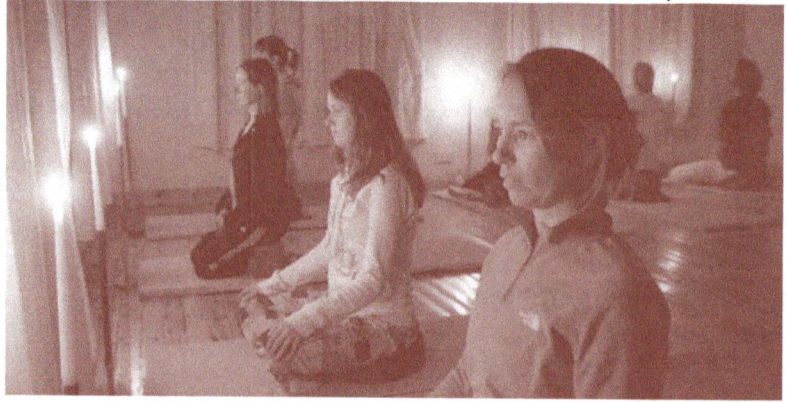

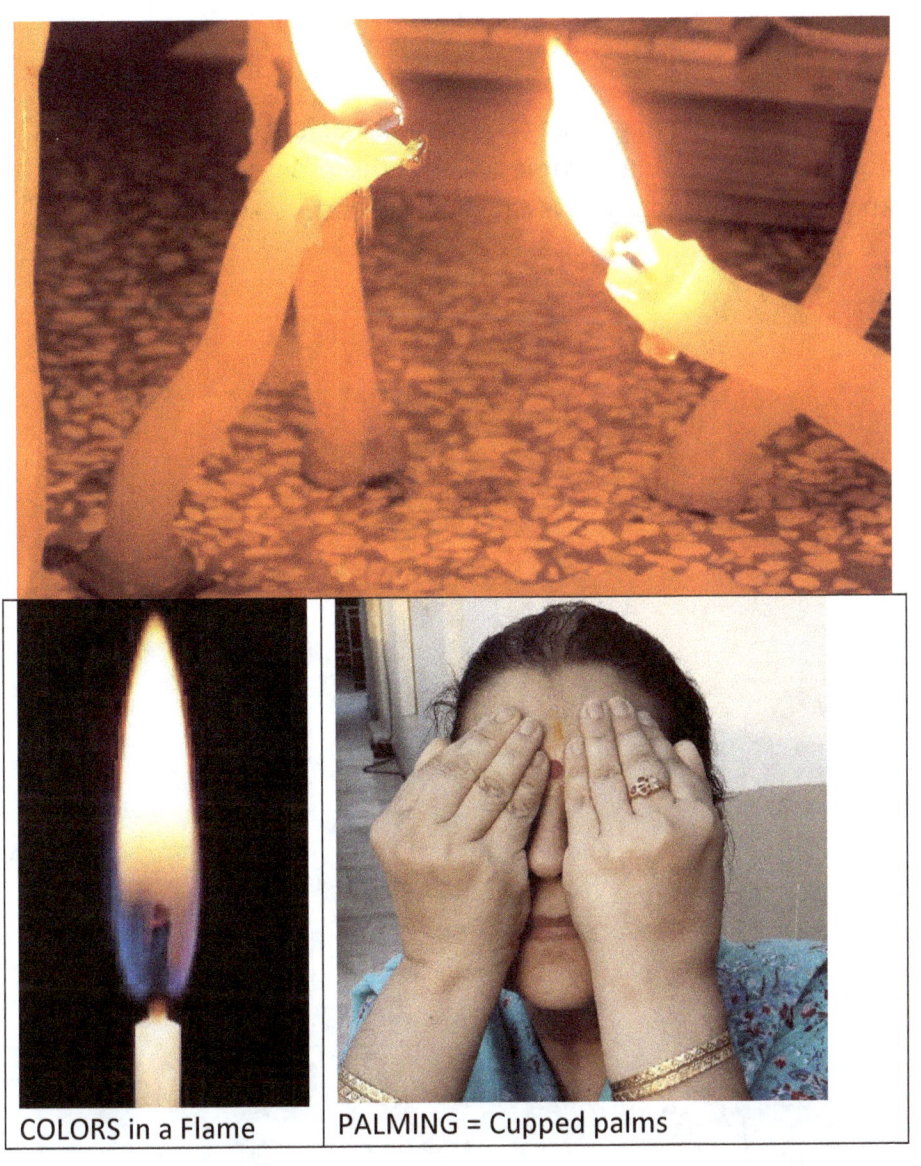

COLORS in a Flame   PALMING = Cupped palms

Ensure that there is no draft in the room and the flame is flicker free. May make the room a bit dark using thick window curtains and switching off ambient lighting.

Palming and Relaxation is a must after Trataka. In palming we cup the hands so that we do not touch the eyes. The eye must be free to blink and move.

Pinhole Text Reading

We read text on a page using the pinhole occluder. Font size that is normally unreadable becomes clear in this process. In that case know that reduced vision is caused by refractive error.

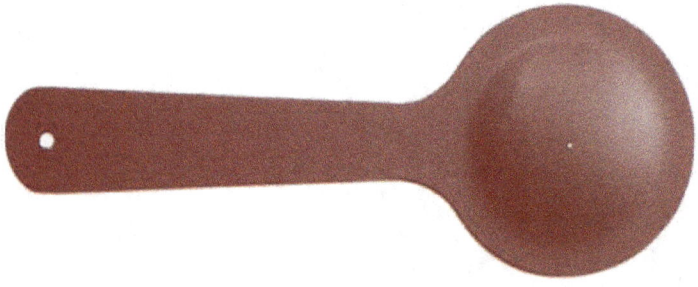

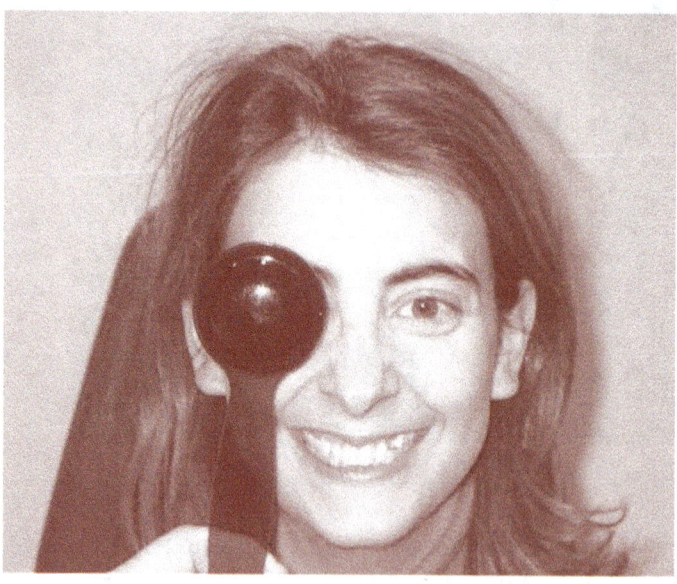

Next Page is a sample text sheet to be used with the pinhole occluder. It contains text in varying font sizes. Close one eye and cover it with the palm. From the other eye, see through the pinhole and try to read each line letter by letter. Note down the smallest font you can read clearly. Repeat with the other eye.

Sukhi bhava! It is an order as well as a blessing. 16

Wherever there is sincerity, people do recognize it. 15

When your intentions are pure & clear, nature supports. 14

The power of spiritual knowledge gives you centeredness. 13

Peace is your very nature. Peace is innate; it cannot leave you. 12

Don't hurt anyone with your speech; for Divine dwells in every heart. 11

You are being fully taken care of. You are being loved dearly. 10

If even the slightest desire to be free has arisen in you, pat yourself on the back, you are very lucky. 8

Look at Events come and go. Both pleasant and unpleasant events come and pass by, leaving you untouched. 7

Deep inside you, observe the intense sensation that creates pain. It flips over and the very sensation assumes a blissful dimension. 6

Do not be feverish about Success. If your aim is clear and you move towards it with patience you shall find unexpected support from all quarters. 5

Steaming with Eucalyptus Oil

- Clean your face thoroughly. You may use Rosewater.
- Use a good quality facial steamer. E.g., https://www.amazon.in/Dr-Trust-Steamer-Vaporizer-Humidifier/dp/B07RM4GKYR/
- Add a drop of virgin eucalyptus oil to the water.
- Use a bath towel over the head to prevent stray breeze.
- Stay at a comfortable distance to avoid overheating.
- Stop after 10 minutes.

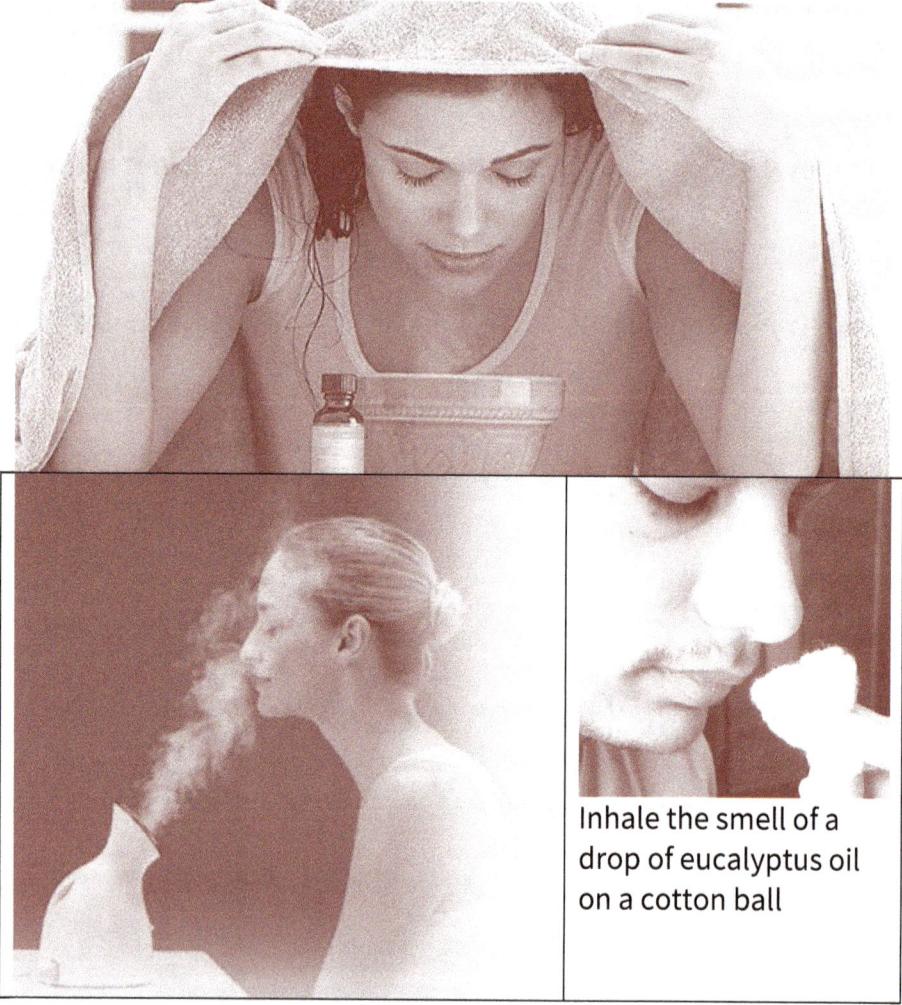

Inhale the smell of a drop of eucalyptus oil on a cotton ball

https://www.amazon.in/NILGIRIS-EUCALYPTUS-ESSENTIAL-OILS-DISTILLERY/dp/B08FFQX743/

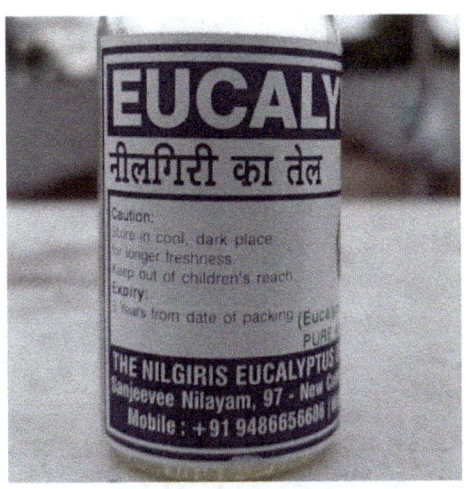

Rosewater Eye Relaxation

After the steaming, lie down on the Yoga mat. Sprinkle rosewater on two pieces of soft tissue paper and cover the eyes with them. Play some relaxing music. (may cover head with a towel).

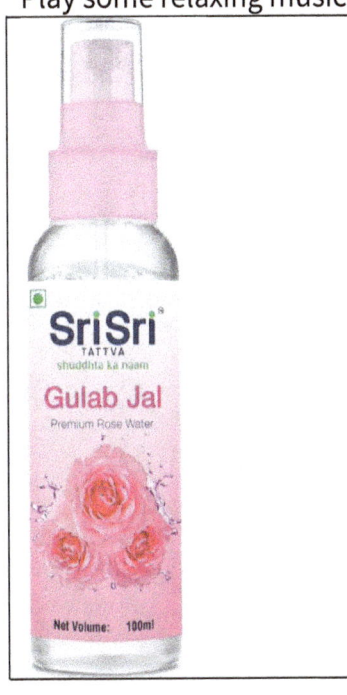
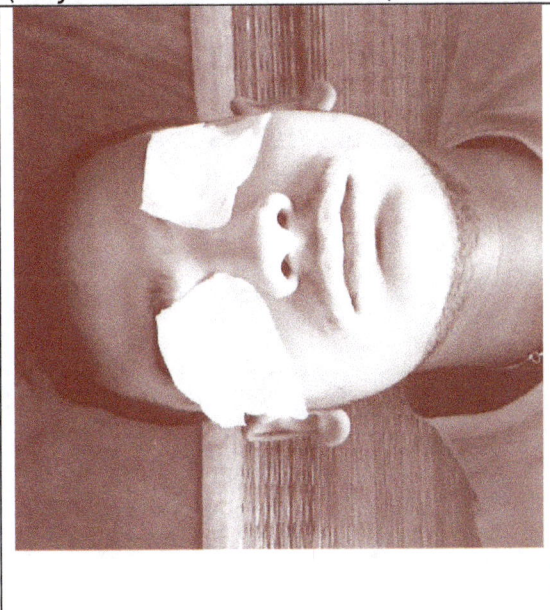

After few minutes remove the tissues (and towel) and lie down in Shavasana for Yoganidra.

Yoganidra

Lie down in Shavasana. Relax the body and loosen the muscles and joints. Take a few deep breaths. Now move the attention slowly from the tips of the toes to the top of the head, stopping for a second at each body part and breathing naturally.

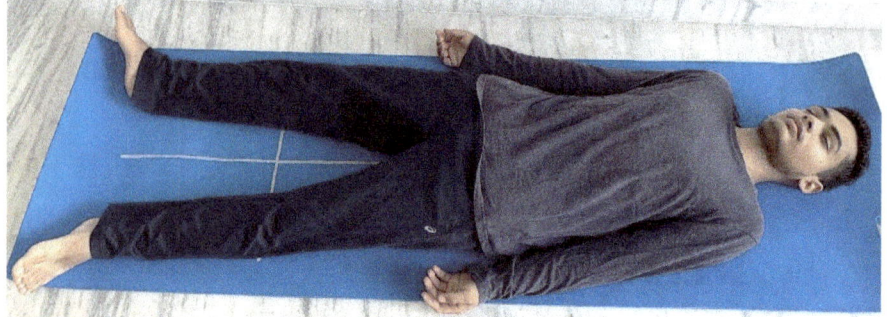

Make a sankalpa for self-betterment, usually to incorporate a virtuous habit or wishing wellness for society at large.

You may use a guided Yoganidra. E.g.
Anandmurti Gurumaa https://gaana.com/song/yog-nidra-hindi
https://www.youtube.com/watch?v=n_ce66a9MV0
Sri Sri https://www.youtube.com/watch?v=HJ5wN5PtwTw

Ashram Experience

Under the able guidance of Dr Padmalochan Jena (founder of the Sri Sri Netra Jyoti, a panchakarma treatment for the eyes) I underwent a 10 days' workshop at Bangalore Ashram in 2016. Initial checkup showed my farsightedness (hyperopia) to be 1.25 which had been since a few years. After the ten days program, the number had dropped to zero and I was spectacles free.

https://www.artofliving.org/in-en/ayurveda/therapies/keep-your-eye-healthy-and-strong-part-1
https://www.srisritattvapanchakarma.com/eye-care/
http://srisrinetrajyoti.blogspot.com/p/3.html
http://www.anandway.com/article/450/Ayurvedic-Eye-Care-at-Sri-Sri-Netra-Jyoti,-Bangalore,-India

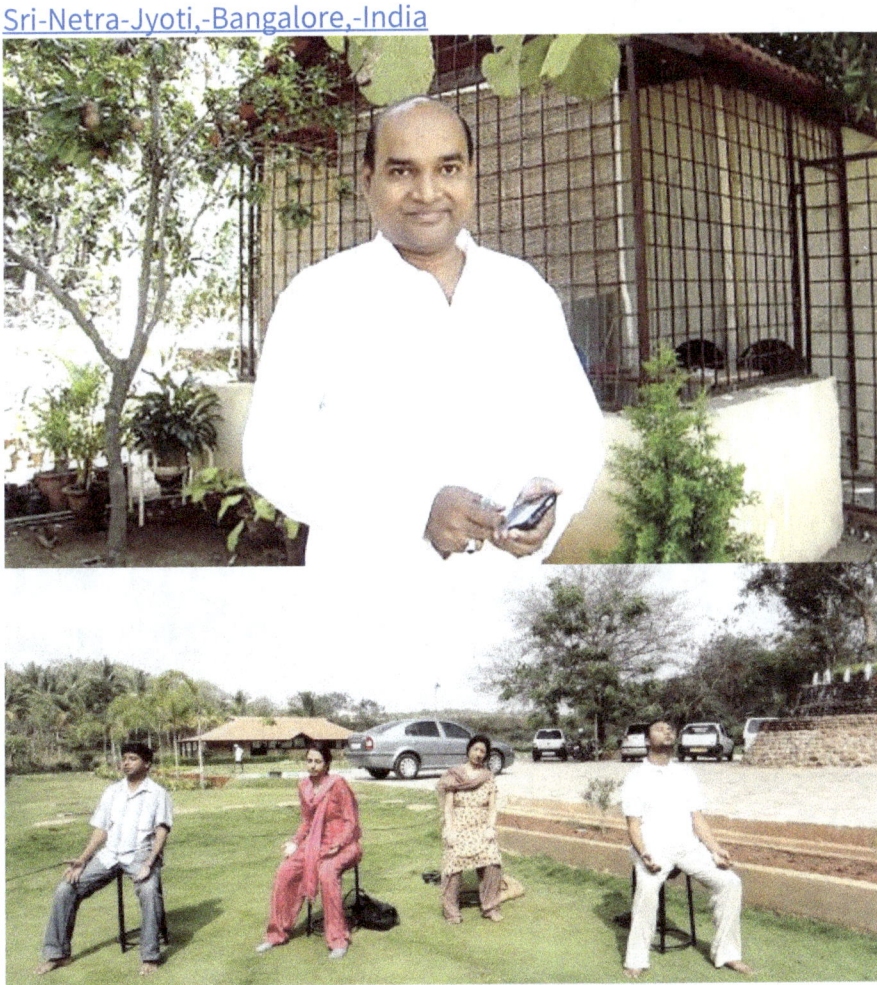

Workshops Facilitated

Patiala June 2016 (two courses, ~100 participants, school children)
Dhuri 2016 (~20 participants)
Malerkotla 2016 (~20 participants)
Mandi Gobindgarh 2016 (~100 participants, school children)
Ludhiana 2017 (morning and evening batches, ~100 participants)
Nabha 2017, 15 to 24 June (~30 participants)
Rajpura 2017, 3-11 June & 21-30 July (~50 participants)
Bathinda 2019, 21 to 30 June (~40 participants, school children)

Also a number of one-to-one individuals have benefitted from these processes.

Known Benefits of Workshop

- Improves Overall Eyesight, whether nearsightedness or farsightedness
- Improves Night Vision, and aids driving confidence and navigating in poor light
- Improves Color Vision, helps us distinguish shades better
- Improves mental abilities for better performance in studies and exams or stressful situations
- Helps ease tired eyes, watery eyes, soreness in eyes
- Helps remove black webs and spots in vision
- Greatly improves teeth and gum health
- Greatly improves hand-eye coordination
- Improves Eye tone and makes eyes more Expressive and Beautiful

Parting get together

At the end of the workshop, we organize a potluck where everyone brings something tasty and nutritious to eat.

First we do a group havan for all-round health, peace and prosperity, followed by singing and sharing experiences amidst bursts of laughter. Then we eat together for caring and sharing in gratefulness.

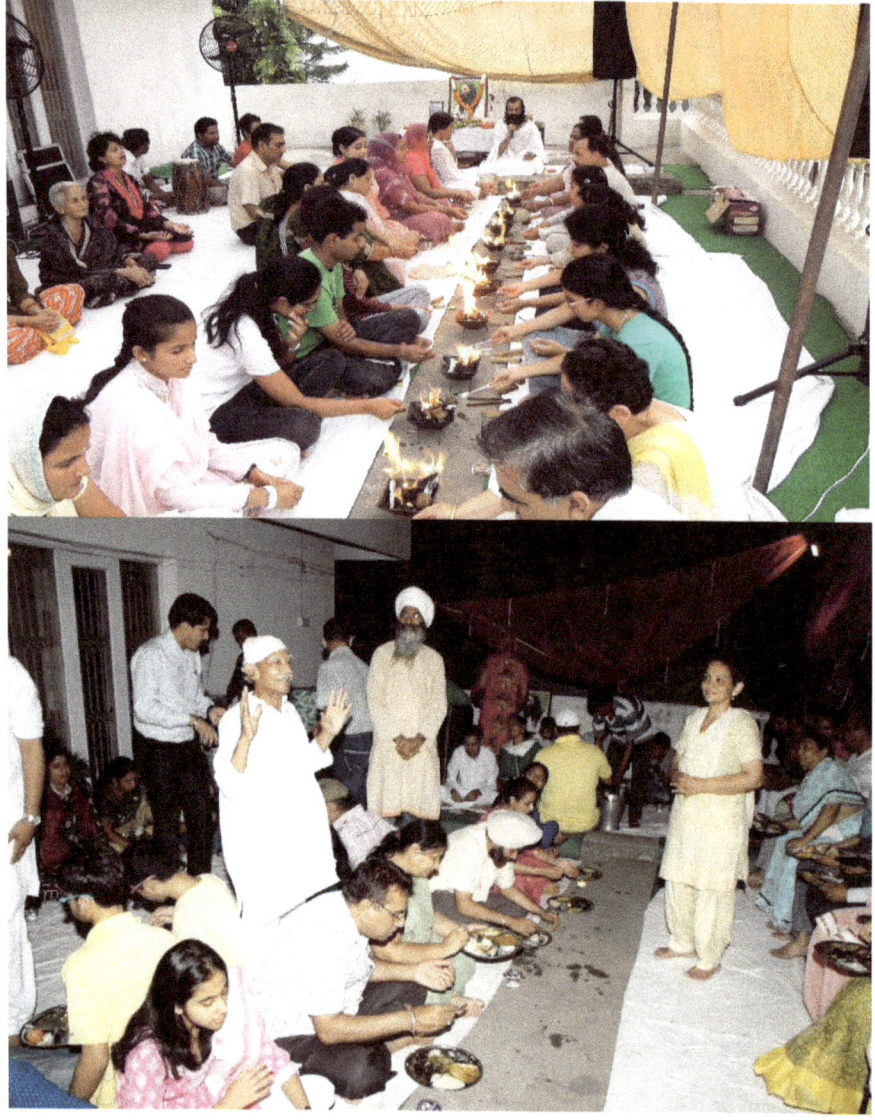

Golden Rule

A golden rule for strong Eyesight is to take a break whenever the eyes feel sleepy, fatigued, or stressed.

Nothing specific, just get up from whatever you were doing and walk around, blink few times, press the eye sockets, wash the eyes, or take a nap.

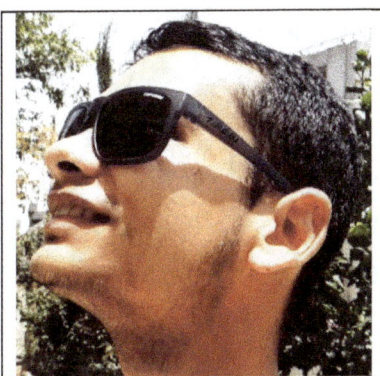 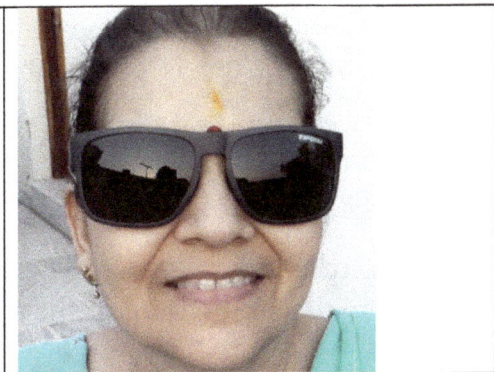

Remember prevention is better than cure.
- Make a habit to wear sunglasses to shade the eyes from harsh sunlight.
- Use an eye mask when the lights are on and you wish to sleep.
- May use anti-glare glasses if you work long on laptop.

https://www.amazon.in/Intellilens%C2%AE-Navigator-Spectacles-Anti-glare-Protection/dp/B07Q7H3PS1/

Process Sequencing

We generally can mix and match the processes depending upon the participants, venue, and ratio of facilitators to participants.

However it is recommended to do the Triphala Eyewash in the beginning and the Rosewater relaxation or Yoganidra at the end.

The sunning exercises should be done in mild sun conditions only, viz. early morning dawn or late evening at dusk. It is recommended to put eyedrops just before doing the sun exercises.

Some processes can be combined to conserve equipment and space. E.g., Skipping and Playing ball and Acupressure walk.

The Snellen Eye Chart check can be done once at the start of the course and then again towards the end, on the 9th day.

Process Regularity

Some processes work best when done daily. Some others can be done every few days.

Triphala Eyewash, Sunning, Candlelight gaze, Coconut oil massage, Dental hygiene, and rosewater relaxation should be done daily.

Active sports, Aromatherapy, Pinhole chart reading, Steam Inhalation, Marma points stimulation can be done every few days.

Yoga and Meditation and Pranayama is a golden rule that works wonders and must be done with reverence in a loving space.

List of Items

A general list of items that are used in the Netra Jyoti workshop.
- Triphala powder (eyewash preparation)
- Neem or babool datun
- Dant Manjan (tooth powder)
- Eyedrops & eyecups (or diwali diyas)
- Candle, candle stand, matches
- Pinhole occluder and a printed page of varying font sizes
- Snellen Eye charts to paste on wall
- Tennis ball (any soft ball) and Skipping Rope
- Carrot Juice, Soaked Almonds (something nutritious & tasty)
- Coconut oil (cold pressed virgin oil)
- Rose water (pure and authentic)
- Tissue paper box and Hand towel
- Eucalyptus oil (pure and natural) and Steamer for inhalation
- Acupressure mat or slippers
- Philips comptalux bulb (high wattage incandescent lamp)
- Yoga mat
- Facility with clear open sunlight space
- Facility with washbasin or running water
- Hall to enable lying down and Yoga for participants
- Music system (soft music for keeping time)

Alphabetical List of Terms

Term	See Topic
Aromatherapy	Aroma for Improved Smell
Asana	Asana for Vision
Ball Playing	Tennis Ball Playing
Candlelight	Candle Light Trataka
Dant Manjan	Datun Dant Manjan
Datun	Datun Dant Manjan
Diet	Nutrition Watch
Eyecup	Triphala Eyewash
Eyedrops	Eyedrops for Lubrication
Eye mask	Golden Rule
Eyewash	Triphala Eyewash
Meditation	Meditation
Moon gazing	Moon and Stars Gazing
Occluder	Pinhole Text Reading
Oil Massage	Coconut Oil Massage
Oral hygiene	Datun Dant Manjan
Palming	Candle Light Trataka
Pinhole	Pinhole Text Reading
Pranayama	Pranayama for Vision
Random Act	Participant's Random Act
Rosewater	Rosewater Eye Relaxation
Sandal paste	Applying Sandal paste
Sankalpa	Participant's Sankalpa
Skipping	Skipping
Snellen Eye Chart	Snellen Eye Chart
Stars gazing	Moon and Stars Gazing
Sunglasses	Golden Rule
Sunning	Sun Exercises
Trataka	Candle Light Trataka
Triphala	Triphala Eyewash
Tumbling E Chart	Tumbling E Chart
Yoganidra	Yoganidra

References

Author	Title	Ed.	Year	Publisher
W H Bates	Better Eyesight Without Glasses	1st	1943	Henry Holt & Co. Inc., New York
https://www.amazon.in/Better-Eyesight-Without-Glasses-Bates/dp/812220709X/				
Meir Schneider	Vision for Life: Ten Steps to Natural Eyesight Improvement	1st	2016	North Atlantic Books, Berkeley, California
https://www.amazon.in/Vision-Life-Natural-Eyesight-Improvement/dp/0369313828/				
Bruce Fife	Stop Vision Loss Now	1st	2018	Piccadilly Books, Ltd., Colorado
https://www.amazon.in/Stop-Vision-Loss-Large-Print/dp/1533116709/				
Esther van der Werf	Optimal Eyesight: How to restore and retain great vision	1st	2019	Visions of Joy, California
https://www.amazon.in/Optimal-Eyesight-restore-retain-vision-ebook/dp/B08PPD1LKJ/				
Marc Grossman & Michael Edson	Natural Eye Care: Your Guide to Healthy Vision and Healing	1st	2019	Natural Eye Care, Inc., New York
https://www.amazon.in/Natural-Eye-Care-Healthy-Healing-ebook/dp/B07V1WZ8VT				

Epilogue

Your EYES are repairable. YOU can take the responsibility.

Brilliant vision can be achieved. Go for it with confidence.

सर्वे भवन्तु सुखिनः । सर्वे सन्तु निरामयाः ।

सर्वे भद्राणि पश्यन्तु । मा कश्चिद् दुःख भाग्भवेत् ॥

ॐ शान्तिः शान्तिः शान्तिः ॥

When faith has blossomed in life, Every step is led by the Divine.
Sri Sri Ravi Shankar

Om Namah Shivaya

जय गुरुदेव

www.ingramcontent.com/pod-product-compliance
Lightning Source LLC
LaVergne TN
LVHW021337080526
838202LV00004B/206